MEDICAL LICENSURE AND DISCIPLINE IN THE UNITED STATES

MEDICAL LICENSURE AND DISCIPLINE IN THE UNITED STATES

ROBERT C. DERBYSHIRE, M.D.

THE JOHNS HOPKINS PRESS
BALTIMORE AND LONDON

FOR KIT

CONTENTS

LIST OF TABLES

CONTENTS

PREFACE

In 1967 the first definitive book on the history of medical licensing in America appeared. Written by Richard Harrison Shryock, an eminent medical historian, and entitled *Medical Licensing in America, 1650-1965* (The Johns Hopkins Press), it is an exhaustive study of the evolution of the licensing system as we know it today. Shryock presents the history of American licensure against the background of procedures as they evolved in other countries, notably Great Britain and some of the European nations.

The present volume is designed to take up where Dr. Shryock left off, and to present an analysis of the practical aspects of medical licensure in America today. In this volume, any reference to the history of licensing is made solely to provide background; for a full account of the history of licensing, I advise the reader to consult Dr. Shryock's authoritative work.

Today from all sides we hear expressions of alarm over the critical shortage of medical manpower in America. Many of the apparent shortages are due to faulty distribution of physicians rather than lack of them. Nevertheless the growing social consciousness of the American people, along with existing and planned government medical programs such as Medicare, will create a demand for increasing numbers of physicians; therefore, the licensing authorities will find themselves torn between the persistent demands of the public for more physicians and their own duty to uphold standards of medical practice.

Although for many years it has been necessary for a physician to obtain a license before beginning the practice of medicine, many people, particularly medical educators, have begun to question the licensing methods used today. One argument which one frequently hears sounds something like this: Following the Flexner Report in 1910 medical education was rapidly improved and practically all of the "diploma mills" were closed. Later, due to the efforts of the American Medical Association (A.M.A.) and the Association of American Medical Colleges, the so called "C" grade schools were eliminated so that today all of the medical schools in the United States and Canada are approved. Therefore, why must a graduate of one of these approved schools, who has already passed rigorous examinations, be subjected to an outside evaluation of his education by a series of state medical board examinations which are of inferior quality and are administered by examiners, many of whom are far removed from medical education?

But even the most vociferous opponents of the present system of licensure admit that there must be control of the quality of physicians and that this control could be weakened by insistent demands for more physicians. This was exemplified by a recent congressional hearing in which the chairman expressed concern over the fact that there is too little control over poorly trained foreign graduates who are practicing in many of the state hospitals today.

The arguments of the advocates of the present system of licensing may be summed up as follows: 1. Licensure is strictly a function of the state governments; therefore, because of their rigid adherence to the doctrine of states' rights they resent any suggestion that there is room for improvement of their procedures. 2. The medical license entitles the licensee to practice as a physician and surgeon, presumably as a general practitioner, not as a specialist or as a scientist or educator. Hence, the members of boards of medical examiners, the majority of whom are practicing physicians, are best able to judge the fitness of an individual to embark upon a career in clinical medicine. Despite the decline in the prestige and numbers of general practitioners, all boards of medical examiners are in essence licensing just this type of physician and requiring him to possess detailed knowledge in a large number of fields.

The licensing authorities lose sight of the fact that no medical school presents a course in that nebulous subject, "General Practice," and of the fact that all of the medical courses are taught by specialists.* 3. Although the authorities are well aware of the ever increasing trend towards specialization, they believe that no matter how specialized a person has become, a doctor is essentially a doctor, and that even a specialist in such a limited field as ophthalmology should be well versed in the rudiments of general medicine. That this argument has some validity was born out by my own observation of an ophthalmologist whose patient developed cardiac arrest during a so-called "minor" eye operation. This doctor's medical horizon was not limited to the eyes; he reacted promptly to the emergency and put into practice his knowledge of resuscitative methods, thus saving the life of the patient.

Today some balance is needed in medicine and its accompanying licensure requirements. If physicians were licensed by the states strictly as specialists there would be a danger that medical education would degenerate into a series of trade schools. On the other hand, no doctor, particularly a specialist, should be expected to be expert in every branch of medicine. That some balance is in sight is attested to by the broad type of multidisciplinary questions now being asked by the National Board of Medical Examiners and the weight placed upon clinical competence testing by the Federation Licensing Examination, described in the text.

Medical discipline, the other important responsibility of the boards of medical examiners also presents difficult problems. Due to their ethical ideals, most members of the medical profession believe that they should be the sole judges of the conduct of their fellows and that they alone should police their ranks. That many members of the general public are convinced that the medical profession is not doing an adequate job of self-policing is evidenced by growing public clamor

---

* Recently, however, Governor Nelson Rockefeller of New York signed a bill requiring each state medical school to form a department of general practice under the direction of a general practitioner. (See *J.A.M.A.* 208:1980, June 16, 1969.)

against physicians, the increasing tendency of federal and state legislative bodies to investigate the conduct of the profession, and the recent rash of books which denigrate the physician.

In a study of professional incompetence I pointed out that between 1960 and 1965 more than 1,000 definitive disciplinary actions had been taken against physicians by the boards of medical examiners. Many of these were because of professional incompetence. Critics have said that this is not a significantly high number. But if one makes a modest estimate that each one of these physicians treats an average of 800 new patients every year, this means that 800,000 people have fallen into the hands of unscrupulous or incompetent physicians during the five-year period. Viewed in this light the "insignificant" figure assumes important proportions.

So far I have mentioned only a few of the problems confronting medical licensure boards today. There are many more. Thoughtful members of the general public, as well as legislators, are with increasing frequency questioning the present methods of licensure. For example, some ask, "Are the boards of medical examiners solely devoted to the welfare of the public? Or, are the boards principally concerned with the protection of the interests of the medical profession and in eliminating competition?"

Since there are as many procedures for licensing and discipline of the medical profession as there are states, a study of all of the laws will force one to answer "yes and no" to both of the above questions.

As a result of many years of observing medical licensing and discipline in America I have concluded that there is no system. My criticism is similar to that of the people who say that there is no system for the delivery of medical care to the people of America. There are so many variable laws and regulations concerning both initial licensure and discipline of physicians that for all practical purposes the United States is composed of a group of tightly organized kingdoms.

In this book I have analyzed the various components of the medical licensure establishment as it exists today. In studying the medical practice laws I have found many inconsistencies and, although complete uniformity is not necessarily essential, it is surprising that we find in a field such as medicine with world-wide applications, that its practice is governed by so many different laws and regulations in the individual states of this country. I have devoted considerable space to the disciplinary aspects of licensure. Without intending to excuse the boards of medical examiners for possible laxity in their avowed purpose of protecting the public against wrongdoers, I have presented some of the problems with which they must contend. The members of examining boards have learned that under any circumstance the administration of justice is not a simple matter.

There may be great changes in medical licensure in the future. Meanwhile this volume is intended to present a fair and accurate picture of the whole field of medical licensure in the United States in the year 1969. No one can deny that many improvements in medical licensure and discipline are urgently needed. However, it is difficult to suggest improvements if one is unfamiliar with the defects of the present system. I hope a dispassionate analysis of the situation, regardless of how much it might annoy adherents to the status quo, will help create some order out of the nationwide chaos of medical licensure today.

Since the material for this book was gathered over a period of several years from a number of different sources, it is impossible to recognize everyone who has contributed. I am grateful to the many members of state boards of medical examiners and of the National Board for stimulating me by means of free exchange of ideas. I am particularly indebted to the secretaries of the state boards who have so promptly and graciously replied to the questionnaires upon which some of the studies cited in this volume are based.

To certain individuals I extend special thanks: To John P. Hubbard, M.D., for supplying me with much material for the chapter on the National Board of Medical Examiners; to Arthur W. Wright, M.D., Lois Hoffman, and E. E. F. von Helms for reading parts of the manuscript and for their suggestions. I am also indebted to H. Doyle Taylor and Oliver Field

MEDICAL LICENSURE AND DISCIPLINE IN THE UNITED STATES

CHAPTER ONE

THE HISTORICAL BACKGROUND OF MEDICAL
LICENSURE IN THE UNITED STATES

Familiarity with early methods of licensure in Europe is necessary to an understanding of the process as it has developed in America. According to Sigerist (1935), medical licensure as an institution became general in Europe during the Middle Ages. While surgeons were generally regarded as craftsmen and were members of guilds, physicians were not craftsmen and their licensing bodies became the medical faculties of the universities. The first faculty to license physicians was that of Salerno, early in the 13th century.

However, during this period surgeons were not completely uncontrolled; they were trained by an elaborate system of apprenticeship. They were required to serve from two to three years with a master, followed by four to six years as journeymen. To become masters they had to pass strict examinations. In sparsely settled areas with insufficient numbers of surgeons for the formation of their own guilds, they joined the guild of blacksmiths; this relationship was based upon the fact that surgeons could and did make their own instruments.

Frederick II, the German emperor who had been elected king of Sicily, wrote the first medical practice law. Farsighted in its requirements, it provided for examination under a regular teacher of medicine at Salerno and for punishment for violation of the law by confiscation of the goods of the offender and a year in prison. Moreover, the law set forth educational standards in the form of three full years devoted to the study of logic. The statute further required that, "after having spent five years in study, he [the physician] shall not practice medicine until he has during a full year devoted himself to medical practice with advice and under the direction of an experienced physician" (Walsh, 1935). Thus the code of Frederick II, promulgated in the 13th century, not only set educational requirements for physicians but also provided for a sort of internship or a minimal period of postgraduate training. Furthermore, the code set fees, required free care for the poor, regulated ethical conduct and, with great wisdom, forbade a physician to own an apothecary's shop.

By 1283 laws similar to those of Frederick II existed in Spain and could be found in Germany by 1347 and in Naples in 1356 (Turner, 1954).

Not until 1511 did England provide for the licensure of physicians (Shindell, 1965). In that year provision was made for an examination to be administered by the bishop of the diocese in which the physician wished to practice. A few years later, in 1518, the system was changed to one of self-regulation by the profession when a charter was granted to the Royal College of Physicians; Parliament confirmed the charter in 1522.

By the time the colonies in America had become well established and some even had their own universities, the necessity for the licensing of physicians had long been recognized in England; but, strangely, the regulations had not spread to the new world and Parliament had not made any effort to regulate the practice of medicine here. The earliest law for control of the medical profession in America was drawn up in Virginia in 1639. This provided for the regulation of the fees of physicians and was apparently precipitated by the belief of the planters that they were being overcharged for the treatment of their slaves. The preamble of the act stated in part, "Whereas by the ninth act of assembly held the 21st of October, 1639, consideration being had and taken of the immoderate and excessive rates and prices expected by practitioners in physick and chirurgy, and the complaints made to the Assembly of the bad consequences thereof, it so happening through the said intolerable exactions that the hearts of divers masters were hardened to suffer their servants to perish for want of fit means and applications than by seeking relief to fall into the hands of griping and avaricious men" (from

Bierring, 1924). The act provided for redress in the courts for overcharging.

In 1736 the Virginia Assembly, still troubled by the economic problems of medical practice, passed "An Act regulating fees and accounts of practitioners in physic." This set forth a definite fee schedule and pointed out that the education of most medical practitioners had been obtained only through apprenticeships. But the fee schedules differentiated between them and those "who have studied physic in any universities and taken a degree therein," the latter being allowed to charge higher fees.

As early as 1649 an attempt was made to regulate the practice of medicine in Massachusetts. Although the act referred to restraints upon unskilled and unethical practices, it was so vague as to be unenforceable. The ineffectiveness of regulation of medical practice in Massachusetts during this period is attested to by a letter to the *Boston Weekly Newsletter*, quoted by Seybold (1930), in which the writer prayed for legislation that "would exterminate the shoemakers, weavers, and almanack makers who are practicing medicine in the Province of Massachusetts." The writer further stated that, while in England physicians were examined for licensure by the College of Physicians, there were no laws against quacks in Massachusetts.

Meanwhile, the apprentice system for education of physicians in the colonies continued to prevail. After the student had completed his apprenticeship his preceptor was the sole authority for admitting him to practice, the only legal requirement being that the physician's application be certified to the court where he was registered.

American citizens continued to deplore the state of medicine and stressed the necessity for effective regulation of the profession. For example, Shryock (1967) quotes William Smith, who said in 1757, "Few physicians among us are eminent for their skill. Quacks abound like locusts in Egypt. This is less to be wondered at as the profession is under no kind of regulation. Any man at his pleasure sets up for physician, apothecary and chirurgeon." The first colonial act requiring a licensing examination was passed in 1760 and applied

3

only to N. Y. City (Shindell, 1965). This provided for a non-medical board of medical examiners consisting of "one of His Majesty's Council, the judges of the supreme court, the King's Attorney General, and the Mayor of the City of New York, or any three of them." These people examined candidates for medical practice and penalties were provided for practice without a license. This was followed in 1762 by a similar statute applying to the whole colony of New Jersey. This law vested authority in the New Jersey Medical Society. In 1773 Connecticut adopted a different approach and required a license before one could collect money for medical services. Presumably anyone could provide medical services if he received no compensation. This principle survives today in several of the states whose statutes defining the practice of medicine stipulate as part of the definition the charging of a fee either directly or indirectly. But not until 1792 did Connecticut follow the lead of New Jersey and authorize the medical society to examine the qualifications of medical practitioners. Meanwhile, Massachusetts and New Hampshire had taken similar action in 1781 and 1791 respectively.

In 1794 the first medical practice act resembling modern American laws was introduced in the Pennsylvania legislature. This was the first attempt to prescribe educational requirements and to require the candidate to present a diploma from a university or college conferring the degree of Doctor or Bachelor of Medicine, or to pass an examination given by a committee composed entirely of physicians. It also provided for reciprocity with other states. However, the bill was tabled by the legislature (Bierring, 1924).

In 1798 the Maryland Legislature passed "An Act to establish and incorporate a medical and chirurgical faculty." It also provided for the appointment of 12 persons "who shall be styled the Medical Board of Examiners for the State of Maryland." Its principal functions were defined as the examination of candidates who wished to practice medicine and to issue them licenses. But apparently the citizens of Maryland eventually found the law too restrictive for, in 1838, the legislature repudiated it and passed an act making it lawful for "each and

4

every person being a citizen of this state to charge and receive compensation for their services and medicine the same as physicians." This situation prevailed until 1892 when the legislature passed a new medical practice act which provided for two boards, one representing the Medical and Chirurgical Faculty, the other the Maryland State Homeopathic Society. There were 20 homeopathic schools in the United States at the time. This law was to remain in effect for more than 60 years and it was not until 1954 that the homeopathic board was abolished by law (Gundry, 1958).

Meanwhile, in Europe, Germany had taken the lead in eliminating second class medical training programs. Prussia instituted the requirement of uniform educational standards in 1852 and its example was soon followed by other German principalities. The new laws required the same state examinations and licenses for all physicians. Says Shryock (1967), "Appeals for medical reform were also voiced at the same time, in the United Kingdom and in the United States; but effective response was delayed in both of these countries—apparently in part, because of the Anglo-Saxon preference for voluntary regulation."

In the United States, by 1830, medical societies had been founded in many of the states. All of them advocated examinations and licensing of physicians. In most cases the legislatures responded by passing licensing laws. These laws were all state-wide in coverage but varied widely in other respects from the establishment of state boards to the granting of licensing power to state medical societies. Moreover, the seat of authority varied from one central body to boards or censors chosen by counties or districts.

Soon the question of licensure by schools arose. This was because the authorities in Massachusetts were impressed by the superior grades of graduates of Harvard in the examinations. Therefore, it was decided that either the Harvard diploma or examination by the medical society could qualify a candidate for practice in Massachusetts. Variations of the plan spread to some other states so that by the early 1800's in practically all of the states candidates for licensure were allowed to practice after they had passed examinations either within their schools or before state boards or medical societies.

But the early promise of medical practice laws to protect the public was not fulfilled and, from 1820 to 1870 licensing requirements steadily deteriorated, due largely to the acceptance of medical degrees as superior licenses. This encouraged the formation of many new inferior schools. Then, as now, some legislatures were sympathetic towards quacks and cultists and readily granted them charters for their schools. By 1845 at least eight states had no licensing requirements at all and some 10 others had repealed earlier regulations. The rapid development of the country in the nineteenth century created a great neeed for physicians with the result that many new schools, mostly inferior ones, were founded (Sigerist, 1935). The licenses granted by such schools meant little. Said Sigerist, "At the time of the Civil War conditions were chaotic; but after the war the readjustment followed rapidly. As the medical schools could not be trusted, the states, or some agencies representing the states, had to take over the control of medical practice. From 1873 on, beginning in Texas, state boards of medical examiners were established, and by 1895 nearly all of the states had such institutions. Everyone knows what a fundamental part these boards have played in the reorganization of medicine in this country."

The part played by the American Medical Association must also be considered. Although the elevation of educational standards was the avowed primary goal of the American Medical Association from its founding in 1846, it could make little progress because many of its members had vested interests in inferior medical colleges and consequently they blocked attempts at reform by state legislatures. But some of the state medical societies had higher ideals. For example, as early as 1839 the New York Medical Society had objected to the combination of teaching and licensing. Moreover, the plans for founding the American Medical Association were made in response to a call from the New York Society which protested the practice of professors licensing their own students, particularly when the latter might expect such a reward in return for fees (Shryock, 1967). N. S. Davis, in his presidential address to the American Medical Association in 1883, announced the following goals: 1. Premedical academic requirements. 2. Minimal time in medical school and hospital training. 3. State boards to provide licensing examinations and the strengthening of professional societies to attain these ends. He added, "The vital point is to take this power [licensing] away from the schools."

In the early 1880's public health agencies were utilized by some states as examining authorities. Notable was the Illinois Board of Health which was given authority to keep a registry of recognized doctors. Later the board prepared a list of medical schools in good standing. Its criteria were essentially those of N. S. Davis. This was the precursor of the idea of approving medical schools which was adopted by the American Medical Association 10 years later.

Although Texas passed the first modern medical practice act (1873), it remained for the West Virginia law, passed in 1881, to provide firm legal precedent for medical licensure. West Virginia's law was challenged in the United States Supreme Court in 1889 and was upheld as a valid exercise of the police powers of the state. Both of these early laws provided specifically for the administration of examinations for the purpose of licensing.

According to Waite (1926), the main cause for the origin of state medical examining boards was the rise of cults such as Thompsonianism, the botanics, and eclecticism; these formed their own societies which in some states were granted licensing privileges. This caused such serious contention that in 1835 several states began to pass legislation to take medical licensing away from the medical societies and place it under state boards of medical examiners appointed by the governor. In some states then, as today, the governor was limited in his appointments to a list submitted by the medical society. At the same time the custom of granting exemption to the graduates of university medical schools grew. But in the last half of the nineteenth century, due to the proliferation of inferior schools, all candidates in every state were required to pass the state board examinations.

By 1895, when all of the existing states had developed legal procedures for the examination and licensure of physicians, the state boards were considered by some reformers as the most important agencies for the elevation of medical education and standards. Flexner in 1910, called the state boards "instruments through which the reconstruction of medical education will be largely effected" (Flexner, 1910). Before that, in 1888, Osler felt convinced that "the future of medical education in this country lies largely in the establishment of state boards such as exist in Virginia, North Carolina, and Minnesota, which shall (1) control the entrance examination, (2) regulate the curriculum, and (3) grant the license to practice" (quoted by Bierring, 1945). (The reason for Osler's later change of attitude is discussed in another chapter.) After the publication of the Flexner Report, further changes and improvements were made in the existing medical practice laws. Later, Turner (1954) reminded the boards that licensing by a state is essentially a guarantee of the knowledge, education and skill of a physician; a state board assumes this responsibility when it licenses physicians either by examination or endorsement.

Although we like to say that the introduction of "modern" medical practice acts began in the nineteenth century and that they were improved after 1910, with the increasing mobility of the physician population another problem arose, namely that of interstate endorsement and reciprocity of licenses. Certain boards, because of their strict requirements, refused to approve physicians licensed in other states. In an effort to solve this problem, in 1902, a Confederation of Reciprocity was founded in Chicago to promote interstate acceptance of licenses. Prior to this, in 1891, state examiners had organized the National Confederation of State Examining and Licensing Boards, the purpose of which was to enable the boards to exchange ideas and to plan stricter requirements. In 1912 the two organizations merged to form the Federation of State Medical Boards of the United States which is still in existence (Bierring, 1923). The program of the first meeting of the new organization in Chicago on February 25, 1913 was concerned mainly with the definition of educational requirements and the mechanics of administration of medical practice laws. As early as 1916 one of the principal topics of discussion was the need for a model or uniform practice act; this has been repeatedly brought up since with no progress. Perusal of subsequent programs might provide the reader with wry amusement if he were not concerned by the recurrence of the same old problems year after year with obvious inability of the Federation or anyone else to solve them.

During this century many states have rewritten or amended their medical practice laws; but some of them are still hopelessly antiquated. The legislative process always lags behind progress in medical education with the result that needed innovations are held back by the laws. Many of the changes in the laws have been designed to improve administrative procedures or to correct loopholes in disciplinary sections which have been discovered by clever defense attorneys. Some states have broadened the powers of their boards of medical

Table 1. Some Highlights in the History of Medical Licensure in the United States

1639	–	Virginia passed first act in America to control the medical profession
1760	–	Act passed providing for medical licensing examinations in New York City
1762	–	Act passed providing for medical licensing examinations in colony of New Jersey
1773	–	Connecticut passed act requiring licensing before compensation could be collected for medical services
1873	–	Texas passed first modern medical practice act in the United States
1889	–	West Virginia's medical practice act of 1881 upheld in U.S. Supreme Court as valid exercise of state's police powers
1912	–	Federation of State Medical Boards formed

examiners to include supervision of other branches of the healing arts such as osteopathy, chiropractic, and podiatry. At present there are 21 such composite boards, while the remainder of the boards confine their activities to the licensing and regulation of physicians.

Despite the provision for penalties for violation of many of the earliest medical practice laws, I can find few detailed references to disciplinary procedures in early accounts. But during the past few years, boards of medical examiners have become increasingly involved with the problems of discipline and daily they receive complaints against doctors from both fellow physicians and irate patients. The power to license implies the power to revoke, but despite progressive broadening of disciplinary powers of boards, they are still limited mainly to violations of the letter of the law. However, the boards are gradually accepting greater responsibilities in the field of discipline and most board members realize that they must assume stricter policing powers if the profession is to continue to regulate itself.

As far as original licensure is concerned, the problem has turned almost full cycle. In the beginning the preceptors licensed their students to practice. Later the medical societies assumed the power of licensure; it was then partially taken over by the medical schools. In each case the system failed because abuses in each field caused lowering of standards. This led to the present method of licensure by boards which are agents of the state governments. This system has been in effect for over 70 years and has been generally successful despite the inconsistencies in certain laws, the lack of uniformity of standards, and the capriciousness of some boards. But many people, particularly medical educators, believe that the function of licensing should be returned to the medical schools.

Shryock (1967) points to the divergences of opinion between organized medicine and medical educators. The latter resent the conservative policies of the medical societies and believe that the rigidity of the boards, backed by the medical societies, hamper the schools in their desire to make innovations in their curricula. Shryock cites the report of a committee of the New York Academy of Medicine in 1947 which said in part, "Licensure by state boards was highly desirable when the standards observed in most schools were very low. . . . Now that relatively high standards are maintained in most schools, it is desirable to return the licensing power to them in order that they may be free to experiment with the curriculum."

The American Medical Association now seems to share the views of the educators concerning the desirability of restoring the licensing function to the schools. Recently Dr. Milford Rouse, president of the American Medical Association, said, "I believe the time has come to consider whether the state medical examining boards really need to require medical graduates to sit for three days writing answers to examination questions that offer few clues to a physician's competence to practice medicine" (Rouse, 1968). Dr. Rouse asked why the boards, having satisfied themselves as to the moral qualifications of an applicant, should not license him on the basis of his medical school transcript. Several prominent educators privately have asked me the same question.

Today many medical schools use an outside agency, the National Board of Medical Examiners, to assess their teaching methods by the administration of examinations of high quality to their students. These schools have a compelling argument in favor of licensure either on the basis of their diplomas or by endorsement of the National Board certificate. But complete return to licensure by the schools is fraught with danger in view of the increasing pressure of the osteopaths for recognition of their schools long before they have been able to elevate their standards to equal those of the approved medical schools. There is also the problem of the foreign graduates whose education in many instances has been inferior to that of the American graduates. Therefore, it could prove disastrous to return to a system of licensure which was long ago found unreliable.

Despite the fact that the National Board of Medical Examiners has for a long time offered a safe and reliable standard for universal licensing, its certificate is still not accepted by some of the states. Until it is universally accepted or until the states recognize some other national standard, the state boards must continue to set their own legal requirements for admission to practice; how much longer some boards will blindly and doggedly insist on defending their states' rights I cannot predict. Meanwhile their artificial and often unreasonable barriers will continue to exact a high cost to advances in medical education and free movement of qualified physicians within the country.

Bibliography

Bierring, W. L. 1923. The First Decade of Federation Activities. *Fed. Bull.** 9:58–62.

————. 1924. The Early Regulation of the Practice of Medicine in America. *Fed. Bull.* 10:295–303.

Flexner, A. 1910. Medical Education in the United States and Canada. The Carnegie Foundation for the Advancement of Teaching. New York: *Bulletin No. 4*.

Gundry, L. P. 1958. History of the Board of Medical Examiners of Maryland. *Maryland Med. J.* 7:5–6.

Osler, W. 1888. Quoted by W. L. Bierring, *Fed. Bull.* 31:162–63.

Rouse, M. O. 1968. Walter L. Bierring Lecture. *Fed. Bull.* 55:70–78.

Seybold, R. E. 1930. Regulation of Practice of Medicine in 18th Century Massachusetts. *New Eng. J. Med.* 202:1067–68.

Shindell, S. 1965. A Survey of the Law of Medical Practice. *J.A.M.A.* 193:601–6.

Shryock, R. H. 1967. *Medical Licensing in America, 1650–1965*. Baltimore: The Johns Hopkins Press.

Sigerist, H. E. 1935. The History of Medical Licensure. *J.A.M.A.* 104:1057.

Turner, E. G. 1954. Measuring Professional Competence. *J.A.M.A.* 154:1203–7.

Waite, F. C. 1926. The Nature of the Responsibility of Medical Licensing Boards. *Fed. Bull.* 12:306–16.

Walsh, J. J. 1935. Earliest Modern Law for Regulation of Practice of Medicine. *Bull. N. Y. Acad. Med.* 11:521–27.

* *Federation Bulletin*, a monthly publication of The Federation of State Medical Boards of the United States, Inc., 1612 Summit Avenue, Fort Worth, Texas 76102.

CHAPTER TWO

MEDICAL PRACTICE LAWS

For a long time physicians have prided themselves on the fact that their profession is self-regulated. But this is true to a limited extent only; self-regulation today is confined to the medical societies which have some disciplinary powers over their members. However, their actions have no force of law. As far as the legal aspects of medical practice are concerned, the profession is anything but self-governing. Although the boards of medical examiners, composed of physicians, ostensibly supervise the practice of medicine, these bodies are controlled in varying degrees by all of the branches of the state governments.

The legislature is the initial body to control the practice of medicine. Not only does it pass the laws which define the methods of control, it also has the power to modify these by periodically amending the medical practice laws. The executive branch of the government plays a part in the regulation of medical practice in that in most states the members of the boards of medical examiners are appointed by the governor, are accountable to him, and can be removed by him for sufficient cause. The boards are also accountable to the judiciary; all of their actions are subject to review by the courts. The boards of medical examiners are administrative bodies with quasi-judicial functions. But the rights of the individual cannot be violated by the boards which have little knowledge of law and many board decisions have been reversed by the courts if they find that they have acted arbitrarily or capriciously or have failed to follow proper procedures.

Contrary to general opinion, the practice of medicine is a privilege and not a right. This was emphasized by the representatives of the boards of medical examiners when the Federation of State Medical Boards of the United States published its "Guide to the Essentials of a Modern Medical Practice Act" (1956). This recommends that a general statement of policy be included in every law. A suggested preamble would read, "Recognizing that the practice of medicine is a *privilege* granted by legislative authority and not a *natural right* of individuals, it is deemed necessary as a matter of policy in the interests of public health, safety and welfare to provide laws and provisions covering the practice of that privilege and its subsequent use, control and regulation to the end that the public shall be properly protected against unprofessional, improper, unauthorized and unqualified practice of medicine and from unprofessional conduct of persons licensed to practice medicine."

Further elaboration of the principle that the practice of medicine is a privilege is provided by Browne (1935), who said in part, "Though many people think that a certificate authorizing them to practice medicine is a grant of a privilege for the peculiar benefit of the holder, nothing can be farther from the theory underlying the granting of a license. The right to practice medicine is a right to protect society, to aid the sick and afflicted, and to assist in the advancement of the health and well-being of those persons who make up the body politic which grants the privilege." Later Browne concedes that once received, the right to practice a profession is a valuable property right, but he emphasizes that it can be taken away not only because of violation of the law under which it was given but it may be summarily rescinded by legislative action. The legislature has the right to say that after a certain date all licenses shall be cancelled. This was actually done in 1838 when the Maryland legislature repudiated a law which it considered too restrictive and passed an art which made it legal for all to practice mediine, an art which remained in force for 54 years (Gundry, 1958)!

The legal control of the practice of medicine was emphasized by Shindell (1966) when he wrote, "While a medical practice act conveys special status on physicians, status is incidental to its primary purpose. Essentially its purpose is to provide a means by which society may exercise formal control over persons designated to minister to its ills." Shindell also points out that the importance of the medical practice act is that it is the public and not the profession who makes the rules. He continues, "Inescapable is the fact that both the privileges and limitations of the profession are in the hands of society."

Early in the history of medical licensure in the United States the constitutionality of a medical practice act was tested in the Supreme Court. In 1882 West Virginia passed a statute which required every medical practitioner to meet one of three standards: 1. He had to be a graduate of a reputable medical college; or 2. He was required to be a practitioner in West Virginia continuously for ten years prior to March 8, 1881; or 3. He must pass an examination prepared by the State Board of Health. One, Dr. Dent, challenged this law in court. He had practiced only since 1876, and he held a diploma from the American Medical Eclectic College of Cincinnati which had been ruled by the Board of Health as not reputable. Dr. Dent did not submit himself for examination by the Board. He was convicted of violating the statute. The Supreme Court of the United States upheld the conviction, noting that the law did not constitute violation of due process as guaranteed by the 14th Amendment (Sears, 1946).

The state, through its medical practice law, not only decides who may practice within its borders but it also defines the conditions under which the physician shall practice. Even after a license has been granted it does not become a permanent property right. The impermanence of a license is emphasized by the fact most states require periodic registration of physicians, many on an annual basis. If a physician fails to meet the registration requirement his license can be suspended and not restored until he has met certain requirements including re-examination in some instances.

In recent years there has been much discussion concerning the advisability of periodic re-examination for recertification. At first shrugged off as an impractical requirement, it is now being considered more and more seriously by many authorities.

The only organization which at present requires its members to keep up to date in medicine by attending a prescribed number of postgraduate courses is the American Academy of General Practice. But re-examination is not part of the requirement. Recently the Oregon Medical Association took steps to impose similar requirements upon its members. A different approach has been adopted by the American College of Physicians, which, on an experimental basis has offered examinations on a voluntary basis to its members. Approximately half of the members took the examinations the first time they were offered. This constitutes an excellent form of self-evaluation as the members' shortcomings are pointed out to them on a confidential basis.

To date, the consensus among both educators and licensing authorities seems to be that postgraduate education should be on a voluntary basis and left to the conscience of the individual. Furthermore the question is often asked, if re-examination for recertification were required, who would administer the examinations? Indeed, it is questionable whether or not the state boards of medical examiners have either the knowledge or ability to re-evaluate their licensees. Should the task be entrusted to the medical schools or possibly to the National Board of Medical Examiners? These questions must remain unanswered for the present.

Re-examination for recertification would require no wholesale changes in the medical practice law. As Shindell (1966) points out, "It certainly is within the power of a state to require re-examination, just as now it is within its power to require examination for initial licensure."

The statutes give the boards of medical examiners the power to revoke licenses as well as to grant them. The grounds for revocation vary widely in the different states but one finds about twelve which are common to all. Although boards are composed of physicians who presumably regulate their own profession, in the case of disciplinary actions, the board members can make only preliminary decisions which can be overturned by the courts and frequently are, sometimes on purely technical grounds. This is particularly true in the case of the malefactor whose crime does not fit neatly into one of the categories of unprofessional and unethical practices enumerated in the law. Complications often arise when the action of the board is based upon the vague term, "unprofessional conduct."

The idea that the medical profession is self-policing is again exploded by the fact that the conduct of disciplinary hearings in all states is carefully prescribed by law. The statutes set forth in detail the procedure which must be followed from the form of the initial notice of contemplated action, through the entire hearing, including the questioning of witnesses and the assurance that the accused be informed that he is entitled to be represented by counsel. The laws require that the findings of fact and the decision of the board be set forth in precise terms. Precautions are taken to protect the rights of the accused. This sometimes results in members of a board emerging from an attempted disciplinary action with a feeling of impotence and frustration. One can find many instances of miscreants who have gone unpunished because of failure of the board to follow the letter of the law. A board composed entirely of physicians can easily be overwhelmed by the legal maneuvers of clever lawyers whose sole intent seems to be to confuse rather than to arrive at the truth. For this reason some boards retain expert legal counsel and heed his advice. While some are ably represented by the members of the staff of the state's attorney general, all too frequently the least experienced man is assigned to the board and there is no continuity of counsel. Therefore, fortunate is the board whose law permits it to employ private counsel.

Many board members are troubled by the multiple duties demanded of them in disciplinary proceedings. They must act as investigators, prosecutors, jurors, and judges. This is indeed an undesirable state of affairs which applies in all states except for those (such as Oregon and California) whose laws provide for the employment of a hearing officer to prepare the case and present it to the board. The fact that the members are often prejudiced in advance of the hearing was brought out in the appeal of the infamous "goat gland specialist," Dr. John R.

Brinkley. In 1930 the Kansas Board of Medical Examiners revoked his license. Brinkley appealed to the court; his most
telling argument was that the board members were prejudiced
against him before the hearing and that some of them had been
active in bringing the complaint against him. The court
agreed that some of the board members had expressed prejudice
and no doubt all were prejudiced. According to Sears, the
court was confronted with the necessity of making a decision
in favor of Brinkley because the only body which could try
him was disqualified by prejudice. In this unhappy dilemma
the Circuit Court of Appeals ruled that Brinkley should not go
"Scott free" and decided that a doctor could not by sensational
publicity disqualify the only body with jurisdiction over him
(Sears, 1946).

The practice of medicine for many years has been regulated
by the states; this policy will not change since the federal
government cannot assume this function without an amendment to the Constitution. Although the medical practice laws
of all of the states presumably have one purpose in common—
to guard the health and welfare of the public by protecting
them against unqualified physicians—the methods of accomplishing this vary widely. In fact, anyone studying the statutes
will find such a wide divergence that he will wonder how any
state can accept the certificate of another. There are so many
areas of disagreement that the medical practice laws, viewed
as a whole, present a veritable patchwork of definitions, administrative methods, and standards.

The staunch advocates of states' rights defend the situation by saying that every state has its own peculiar problems
and that the medical practice laws have been written with
these in mind. But is this really a defensible position? Is the
science of medicine so inexact that uniform standards cannot
be applied throughout the entire country? Is there such diversity in the practice of medicine throughout the states that it
must be governed by such a wide variety of laws? In the current
age of the jet plane and easy communications such parochialism
is unjustifiable. The courts are upholding this view more and
more in malpractice actions. Formerly a physician was held

only to the standards of practice of his community. But recently the courts have decided that such narrow rules no longer apply and that the physician, particularly the specialist, must live up to practices accepted at the national level. This is exemplified by a recent decision of the Supreme Court of West Virginia which permitted a New York ophthalmologist to testify as an expert medical witness regarding the proper treatment of cataract, since the standards for performance of cataract operations are the same throughout the country.

Obviously the state legislative bodies believe that for the protection of the public, before a person can be allowed to practice medicine, he must obtain a license from the board of medical examiners. But there is such disagreement as to methods that the states cannot even concur on a definition of the practice of medicine. There are almost as many definitions as states. In the first place there is wide variation in the number of words required to define what the law proposes to regulate. The longest definition consists of 195 words in contrast to the characteristic Yankee economy of words in the 30-word New Hampshire law. Because of its succinctness it is worth quoting: "Any person shall be regarded as practicing medicine under the meaning of this chapter who shall diagnose, operate on, prescribe for or otherwise treat any human ailment, physical or mental."

In other state laws the definition of the practice of medicine is spelled out in great detail even to the extent of specifying that any one who attaches to his or her name the words or letters, "Dr.," "Doctor," "Professor," "M.D.," or "Healer," is practicing medicine.

Another important point of variation is whether or not payment of a fee is concerned in the practice of medicine. According to the laws of 23 states, to practice medicine (regardless of other parts of the definition) the person must be paid or expect to be paid a fee directly or indirectly. But in two laws, it specifically states that a person is practicing medicine regardless of whether or not compensation is involved. The remaining laws are silent on the question. There is also wide variation in the penalties for practicing without licenses. In some states it is a felony, while in others it is only a misdemeanor.

From many sources come complaints about the difficulty of persuading district attorneys to prosecute people for practicing medicine without licenses. This, of course, has little to do with definitions, but with indifference and possible laziness. However, in one state law there is no specific definition of the practice of medicine so there should be no grounds for criticism of prosecutors there.

Another point upon which there is much variation among the state laws is the standards required for licensure. In 1967 Ruhe, in an attempt to determine whether state licensure laws constituted a serious barrier to innovations in medical education, analysed the medical practice acts of all of the states. He obtained his information both from a study of the statutes and of the regulations of the boards of medical examiners. He found that 42 boards have rules going back as far as the high school level. In 39 states the high school requirements are incorporated in the laws. In general the laws require a high school diploma or graduation from a high school, but, according to Ruhe, "In most instances the requirement is tempered by the phrase 'or its equivalent,' which permits the board to exercise its judgement as to whether the intent of the law has been satisfied." But in two state laws graduation from high school is required without allowance for "equivalence." In no law are the details of the high school curriculum spelled out.

Entirely different is the situation regarding the legal requirements concerning premedical courses. Twenty-nine states specify the necessary amount of college work, while 12 have requirements regarding the details of the curriculum. Two of the laws go so far as to prescribe the length of the required courses. One law states that a candidate for licensure shall have not less than two years or 60 semester hours of college credits, including such courses as may from time to time be prescribed by the board. The capriciousness of some of the boards in deciding the courses that should be included in the college curriculum was emphasized in the recent case of a graduate of a foreign medical school who could not be granted a license because he lacked a course in music appreciation!

In 26 states detailed requirements concerning the amount of medical school work are included in the laws or regulations. Six states require four years of at least 32 weeks each, while eight stipulate four years of at least eight months each. Few statutes specify the content of the medical school courses and these are given in vague terms listing courses in which there must be "adequate instruction."

In 39 states an internship must be completed before a physician can qualify for licensure. Four boards require a rotating internship, one going so far as to specify the exact periods of time which must be served on each service. This requirement is causing consternation among many educators who believe that the internship should be abolished since it is largely a duplication of work performed in medical school. Moreover, they think that students should be allowed to move into their residencies immediately after graduation. But, due to the difficulty of amending medical practice laws, it seems that the internship will not be abolished soon.

The many inconsistencies in the laws concerning specific educational requirements cause much confusion and hamper not only interstate endorsement but constructive experiments in medical education. The insistence of many state boards in setting not only the medical school curriculum but the premedical curriculum, as well, causes me to believe their attitudes can best be expressed by paraphrasing the famous remark of Briand to Lloyd George concerning war—medical education is much too serious a thing to be left to educators.

In all of the medical practice acts there is a requirement that candidates for licensure, with exceptions for endorsement, pass examinations. But the state boards are far from agreement as to the subjects upon which a candidate must be examined in order to determine whether or not he is fit to practice medicine. The laws of 17 states do not specify the subjects in which a candidate must be examined. Presumably these are prescribed by regulations which can be changed at the whim of the boards. In the remaining 34 states whose laws do enumerate the subjects there is wide variation as to what constitutes an adequate examination. I was able to find a total of 59 different required subjects. Many of the states even specify the number of questions on each subject. In addition 15 laws have extra passages permitting the boards to prescribe such additional subjects as they may deem appropriate.

Table 2 shows the ten most popular subjects prescribed by the laws. These laws seem to indicate that the authorities in most of the states believe that a knowledge of physiology, anatomy, pathology, surgery, and chemistry is necessary. Surprising is the fact that medicine is not included in the list. Although many boards do require examinations in medicine, it appears under a variety of designations, such as "Medicine" in nine states, "Practice of Medicine" in six, while in four it is placed with surgery in a subject entitled, "Practice of Medicine and Surgery." In two states the candidate for licensure is examined in the "Theory and Practice of Medicine."

In looking over the vast variety of subjects, many with archaic sounding titles, one wonders whether they were designated by lawmakers who studied 1910 editions of the catalogues of medical schools. For example, one finds such ancient gems as "Symptomatology," "Etiology and Hygiene," "Symptomatology and Therapeutics," and "Materia Medica and Practice."

Table 2. Ten Most Numerous Subjects of Licensing Examinations

Subject	Number of States
Physiology	29
Anatomy	28
Pathology	27
Surgery	27
Chemistry	26
Bacteriology	19
Obstetrics and Gynecology	17
Obstetrics	15
Pediatrics	10
Hygiene	10

Only eight states require examinations in medical jurisprudence, while one examines in legal medicine which is
probably similar.

By studying the laws one also can find certain oddities
among the prescribed subjects of examination. For example,
one state requires an examination in "Urinalysis," another in
"Diagnosis, Including Diseases of the Skin, Nose and
Throat"; not to be outdone, a third state requires the candidate
to pass a subject called "Diseases of the Skin, Eye, Ear, Nose
and Throat and Genitourinary System."

The diversity of prescribed subjects and the many anachronisms found in the list are especially significant in view
of the modern interdisciplinary approach of many medical
schools which prefer not to designate specific subjects but to
build their curricula upon broad general principles which cut
across all disciplines. The National Board of Medical Examiners, aware of this trend, now gives entirely interdisciplinary
examinations. But the Board is able to extract from the computer grades in individual subjects to satisfy the requirements
of state laws.

In the states whose laws specify the examination subjects
there is a wide variety of the number required. One law lists
only four, while another requires 15; the latter state, apparently
to be sure that the field is completely covered, adds "and such
other subjects as deemed necessary by the board."

A glance at Table 3 will reveal that there is complete lack
of consistency regarding passing grades. In 28 states the required grades are not specified in the laws; hence one must
assume that they are set by the rules and regulations of the
board and that they can be changed at will. Most of the 23
laws which do specify passing grades require an average of
75 per cent. However, there is variation in the minimum grades
required, the lowest being 60 per cent. Five laws contain interesting grandfather clauses permitting bonuses for experience
in the practice of medicine. These vary from five per cent for
five years of practice to one per cent for each year of practice
after the first two years. Regarding the latter state, no mathe-
matical wizardry is required to determine that if the candidate

Table 3.   Passing Grades on Examinations

Requirement	Number of States
Not specified in law	28
No grade less than 60, average 75	8
No grade less than 65, average 75	5
No grade less than 70, average 75	3
Grade of 75 in each subject	3
Average of 75	2
Not less than 65 on any subject, average 70	1
Not less than 60, average 70	1

waits long enough he is almost bound to pass. Whether these bonuses are based upon the assumption that experience in practice compensates for academic shortcomings or upon pure political considerations, I cannot say.

The laws vary less widely concerning the personal requirements for licensure. Most prescribe that the candidate must be at least 21 years of age, of good moral character, and a graduate of an approved medical school; on the last requirement there is little agreement as to the methods of approving medical schools. The laws of 26 states specify that the board itself shall approve the schools, while 14 define an approved school as one passed by the Council on Medical Education of the American Medical Association, The Association of American Medical Colleges, or both. Ten laws require graduation from a reputable medical college or a duly chartered college without adding definitions. Two laws state that the schools must be approved by the American Medical Association but reserve for the board the right to approve additional schools. One law goes so far as to require the members of the board to inspect schools periodically.

Mundane matters such as the cost of a medical license are important to a candidate. There is wide variation in the fees required; they range from $20.00 to $100.00 for examinations and from $10.00 to $200.00 for certification by endorsement. Oddly enough, the majority of states charge more for licensure by endorsement than by examination. One would expect the reverse to be true as the administration of examinations is more difficult and time-consuming. A few boards charge graduates of foreign medical schools more than graduates of schools in the United States.

All state laws which permit licensure by endorsement state that this can be permitted only if standards are equal. And how equal can standards be with the wide divergence in passing grades? And what of the states which require examinations not commonly required such as in Medical Jurisprudence? Can they endorse the licenses of states which have no such requirements? Somehow or other they do, although petty quarrels frequently arise between states when a capricious board decides to scrutinize the standards of another; but eventually these difficulties are ironed out only to crop up again elsewhere. At best it is a poor situation.

There is little consistency in methods of examining. Some 16 state boards use examinations furnished by the National Board of Medical Examiners, seven use the Federation Licensing Examination, and a few use a professional testing service. The remainder use questions composed by their own board members. Here again there is lack of uniformity of standards with a mixture of essay and objective examinations.

What are the states doing to improve their laws? Very little, I am afraid. Boards of medical examiners and state medical societies are reluctant to rewrite even hopelessly antiquated laws until they are sure that the political climate is just right—and that time never seems to arrive. Some have learned by bitter experience that their most carefully prepared bills, after being buffeted about in committees and in legislative chambers can emerge unrecognizable because of amendments tacked on by eager but shortsighted legislators. Consequently few states have completely rewritten their laws recently. They usually solve their immediate problems by having an occasional amendment passed; but by this method the medical practice acts turn into inefficiently patched up documents at best.

Notable exceptions to the above generalizations are California, Oregon, Ohio, and Arizona which have passed completely revised medical practice laws during the past five years. Most of the new laws present few real innovations, the current versions being mainly designed to solve house-keeping problems of the boards. But in some cases definite advances have been made in that the provisions for discipline have been greatly strengthened. Notable among these is the tendency of several states, such as Ohio, to require a physician whose license has been inactive to prove to the board by passing an oral or written examination his fitness to resume the practice of medicine. The Ohio law also provides that the board may require an individual to obtain further training and it may also limit the scope or type of practice. Washam (1968), formerly Executive Secretary of the Ohio board, states that these provisions should aid the board in situations where professional competence is at issue.

The most important advance in the strengthening of medical practice acts occurred in California in 1966. Before the new medical practice bill was introduced into the legislature extensive hearings were held by the Senate Fact Finding Committee on Public Health and Safety. These involved the State Medical Association, the Board of Medical Examiners, law enforcement officers, and representatives of the general public. A large volume was required to record the deliberations of the committee; but it makes for exciting reading because of the many thoughtful and constructive views expressed and because it represents a model of cooperation among the agencies concerned.

The revised California statute greatly increases the disciplinary powers of the Board of Medical Examiners. For example, the definition of unprofessional conduct was broadened to include gross negligence, gross incompetence, and gross immorality. The probationary authority of the board was extended to afford better methods of rehabilitation of errant physicians. Because of the large number of physicians appearing before the board for disciplinary reasons, district review committees were formed to assist the board and to prevent long delays in holding hearings.

In California, as elsewhere, the accredited hospitals have

provided adequate safeguards in their bylaws for the protection of their patients. In these hospitals the qualifications and conduct of the members of the staff are specifically defined and, by an elaborate series of committees, the quality of practice is periodically reviewed. But in California, as in some other states, there are many hospitals which are not accredited, their only regulation consisting of inspection by the State Department of Public Health to see that they have met proper sanitation and building safety standards. When a physician, because of incompetency or unprofessional conduct was dropped from the staff of an accredited hospital, he could continue his depredations in the shelter of one of the "fringe" or unaccredited hospitals which are more interested in the revenue brought in by the physician than in his competence or morals. But a provision in the new law might well put a stop to this; under it the board of medical examiners can take action on grounds of unprofessional conduct against a physician who regularly treats patients in a hospital which does not have an established mechanism for periodic review and evaluation of medical care. Furthermore, the law, without mentioning the Joint Commission for the Accreditation of Hospitals, delineates acceptable standards which are similar to those necessary for accreditation.

California, because of its burgeoning population has more than its share of medical problems. The authorities are acutely aware of them and the board of medical examiners continually tries to safeguard the citizens against incompetent and unscrupulous practitioners and charlatans. The recent improvements in the medical practice act are ample evidence that the board's efforts are bearing fruit. The new medical practice law might well serve as a model for all of the other states.

As far as administration of the laws is concerned there is also variety as to types of boards and the jurisdictions under which they function. Twenty-one states and the District of Columbia have composite boards which means that other members of the healing arts are represented on them, such as osteopaths and chiropractors. The other 30 boards are made up solely of M.D.'s. In the District of Columbia and in three

states the boards of medical examiners are under the supervision of Departments of Licensure; in four states the boards
are under the Department of Health; in three they are under the
Department of Education. In the remaining 40 states the boards
are separate, self-governing agencies. Many physicians are
opposed to boards of medical examiners giving up any of their
independence. They believe that the main danger of having
medical boards under a department of licensure is that the
director, who can have dictatorial powers, might be a political
hack with no qualifications for the job. Under such a system,
the director would not be compelled to heed the advice of the
members of the board of medical examiners who are better
qualified to establish policies and to make final decisions.

A real threat to standards is possible in some of the composite boards which, for political reasons, sometimes lower
their passing scores lest too many of the non-M.D. candidates
fail the examinations.

After the special right to practice medicine has been con-
ferred upon the physician in the form of licensure, it is imperative that he realize that this does not permit him to impose his
will upon a patient. Shindell (1965) sounded a note of warning
in this regard when he said, ". . . our Society is characterized
by the principle that each man is capable of independent
judgement and the right to exercise that judgement. When a
physician undertakes to treat a patient, therefore, he can do so
appropriately only with the recognition that our Society holds
that the patient is a free agent and that the physician is essentially an advisor."

The American Medical Association exercises much control
over medical licensure because of its broad influence in the
setting of educational standards, and the Association of
American Medical Colleges exercises an equal influence; the
two organizations together set the standards. And what other
bodies are qualified to do so? Certainly not the boards of
medical examiners, although some of them do attempt to spell
out the curriculum both in the college and in the medical
school. With the almost universal efforts of the medical schools
to improve their curricula, sometimes by making radical

changes, it is not wise for the legislatures, through the boards, to dictate detailed standards of education. Now that there are no more diploma mills or unaccredited medical schools this can be safely left to the experts.

What happens when a medical practice act requires amendments or even complete revision? There is no such thing as a perfect law and experienced members of boards of medical examiners are the first to recognize this. They are the people who first detect weaknesses in their laws and they should initiate action to correct them. But this can be a long and tedious procedure no matter how obvious the defects in the law. The usual procedure is to draw up a preliminary draft with the advice of counsel. Then the help of the state medical society must be sought. The preliminary draft is submitted to the legislative committee for further suggestions. This can constitute a real hurdle because some of the members lack experience in the law. The proposed changes then go to the house of delegates of the medical society which engages in still more discussion. If the draft now emerges in recognizable form and is supported by the medical society, its legislative committee enlists the aid of one or more of the legislators who introduce it. The bill must then go to committees of both houses of the legislature where there is always the danger of undesirable changes being made. An additional danger is that amendments will be made from the floor of either house.

A natural question is, why should the boards, agents of the government, be so concerned over the opinions of the medical societies? There are two answers to this. First, the members of the medical society will be directly affected by changes in the law and should be consulted. Secondly, without the support of the medical societies it is all but impossible to persuade legislatures to act. It is remarkable that anything is accomplished using such a cumbersome system; but if the case is well presented the chances are good that both the medical society and the legislature will be understanding and helpful.

Many medical practice laws are obviously archaic and badly in need of revision, but because even less desirable laws may emerge, board members are reluctant to attempt revisions.

This emphasizes that the medical profession is not self-regulating but is controlled by law; though changes in medical practice laws are initiated by the medical profession, the legislatures have the final word.

As far as the philosophy of medical licensure is concerned, both the legislature and society in general are content to allow the medical profession to regulate itself within certain limitations. They are reluctant to interfere in matters with which they have no expert knowledge. But, as Miller (1934) has pointed out, if society finds that its faith has been abused and "that the benefits of the profession can be better secured and its dangers better guarded against by greater regimentation and government domination, these changes will come in spite of the protests of those who are most professionally conscious."

Shindell (1966) neatly summed up the philosophy of medical licensure when he said, "The importance of the medical practice act in viewing the relationship of the physician to our legal system is to emphasize that it is the public and not the profession who makes the rules. Inescapable is the fact that both the privileges and limitations of the profession are in the hands of society." I am repeatedly struck by the fact that so many physicians regard the acquisition of a license as a formality or as an annoyance to be overcome on their way to practice. Few of them realize the seriousness of the procedure and the fact that they have definite legal as well as moral obligations to the public. Even fewer have the most superficial knowledge of medical practice laws. This is a deficiency which can best be remedied by close cooperation between the boards and the state societies. This cooperation already exists in some states but progress is slow in many others in which the boards of medical examiners seem to operate in a vacuum.

Because of the concern of both the federal government and the public over both medical manpower shortages and the maintenance of uniformly high professional standards, it is high time that the states and their boards of medical examiners correct the hodgepodge of laws and multiple standards lest changes be effected in a manner which will be unpalatable to them.

Bibliography

Browne, L. 1935. Regulation of Professions by the State. *California and Western Med.* 43:119–23.

Federation of State Medical Boards of the United States. 1956. *A Guide to the Essentials of a Modern Medical Practice Act.*

Gundry, L. P. 1958. History of the Board of Medical Examiners of Maryland. *Maryland Med. J.* 7:5–6.

Hundley v. *Martinez.* 158 S.E. 2d 159. (W. Va., Dec. 12, 1967).

Miller, J. 1934. The Philosophy of Professional Licensure. *Fed. Bull.* 20:201–24.

Ruhe, C. H. W. 1967. Are There State Licensure Barriers to Innovations in Medical Education? *Fed. Bull.* 54:146–54.

Sears, K. C. 1946. The Medical Man and the Constitution. *Ann. Intern. Med.* 25:304–23.

Shindell, S. 1965. A Survey of the Law of Medical Practice. *J.A.M.A.* 193:601–6.

———. 1966. *The Law in Medical Practice.* Pittsburgh: University of Pittsburgh Press.

Washam, W. T. 1968. A Step Forward in Ohio. *Fed. Bull.* 55:79–82.

CHAPTER THREE

THE MEMBERS OF STATE BOARDS
OF MEDICAL EXAMINERS

I n "A Guide to the Essentials of a Modern Medical Practice Act," published by the Federation of State Medical Boards of the United States (see Appendix), the first recommendation is that a general statement of policy should introduce an act. Although only six states have chosen to incorporate such preambles in their laws, the principle defining the functions of state boards is worthy of further emphasis. It reads, ". . . it is deemed necessary as a matter of policy in the interests of public health, safety and welfare to provide laws and provisions concerning the granting of that privilege and its subsequent use, control and regulation to the end that the public shall be properly protected against unprofessional, improper, unauthorized and unqualified practice of medicine and from unprofessional conduct by persons licensed to practice medicine."

Protecting the public against the admission of unqualified physicians into their states and insuring that their conduct remains above reproach after admission are indeed awesome responsibilities. These of necessity have fallen upon the boards of medical examiners. Therefore, it is logical to ask what kinds of people accept these responsibilities?

Who are the individual members of state boards of medical examiners? How are they appointed? What qualifications must they have to serve? What educational standards have they met? To answer these and other questions I studied the medical practice laws of all of the 50 states. I also made a survey of pertinent biographical data concerning the members as listed in the American Medical Directory (American Medical Association, 1967).

As one would expect with 50 jurisdictions, there is a wide variety of methods of appointment of members who serve on boards of medical examiners. Although most members are appointed by the governor, the methods of appointment vary. The laws of 12 states merely state that the board members shall be appointed by the governor. In 10 states they are appointed by the governor with the consent of the senate. In 19 states the governor makes the appointments from lists submitted by the state medical associations. The laws of 16 states specifically require the governor to make his appointments from lists of recommended candidates submitted by the state medical association. In three states the governor "may" select members on the recommendation of the medical association, but he is not compelled to do so.

In one state the appointments are made by the governor with the consent of the senate from a list submitted by the medical society. Alabama's law is unique in that it specifies that the Board of Censors of the Medical Association of the State of Alabama shall constitute the board of medical examiners. In two states, Maryland and North Carolina, the board members are selected directly by the medical associations. Therefore, regardless of minor differences the laws of 23 states provide that the medical society shall have a direct voice in the appointment of members.

Other methods of appointment of board members include the following: in Nebraska the members are appointed by the Department of Health; in New York by The Board of Regents of the University of the State of New York (The State Education Department); The Pennsylvania and Illinois boards are under the Board of Education, while in Kentucky and Mississippi the members of the Boards of Health constitute the boards of medical examiners.

I was particularly interested to learn that in 16 states the governor is required to appoint board members from lists submitted by the state medical associations. For many years I have heard muttering from various legal authorities to the effect that this is an unconstitutional usurpation of the appointive powers of the executive. But I can find only one instance in which the legality of the board has been seriously challenged in the court for this reason. This occurred in New Mexico in 1967. The licenses of two doctors were revoked for fraud and deceit in the practice of medicine. As they were not members of the state medical society, their lawyer contended that they were discriminated against because the hearing was held before a board, all of whose members belonged to the medical society and who had been appointed from a list of candidates submitted to the governor by the society. On appeal, while the judge reversed the decision of the board for other reasons, he did not rule that the board members had been appointed illegally. Nevertheless, it is strange that the medical societies can exercise so much influence in the appointment of quasi-judicial boards which are arms of the state governments. And, of course, the influence of the medical societies in the states in which the board members are directly appointed by the medical societies reaches an extreme degree. Moreover, while accurate statistics are not available, it is well known that many past or present officers of medical societies serve on boards. Possibly the reason for their authority not having been challenged is that the aggrieved doctor can appeal to the court, if disciplinary action has been taken against him.

In states having composite boards* in which the law specifies that board members shall be appointed by the governor from lists, it also provides that lists be submitted by other societies in filling vacancies concerning their own members such as osteopaths and rarely chiropractors.

Many members of state medical societies are proud of the fact that they can guide the choice of the governor in his appointments of board members. They claim to have removed politics from the board and that they are in a better position to judge the qualifications of prospective board members than is the governor. They contend he might use his authority to pay off political debts in his appointments rather than to select the

* A composite board is defined as one which licenses other members of the healing arts in addition to M.D.'s, such as osteopaths and sometimes chiropractors.

best people for the positions. But the medical societies ignore the importance of medical politics which often is little above the ward heeler level. In 1963 this was impressed upon the Federation of State Medical Boards of the United States by Pearson when he said, "Let me call your attention to the fact that there is such a thing as medical politics and so the boards, as well as all medical examiners of the boards, have as their duty the administration of the state laws subject to (but we hope not necessarily influenced by) the matter of politics."

The medical societies are by no means always likely to recommend the most highly qualified people for appointment to boards. Frequently they ignore professional and educational attributes, endorsing some faithful political stalwart who has worked his way up in the councils of his society. I know of one case in which the first choice of the governing body of a medical society to fill a vacancy on the board was a graduate of an unapproved medical school; this despite the fact that the law specifically provided that all members must be graduates of approved schools, the definition of which was spelled out. Fortunately an alert executive secretary detected the error thus preventing a serious blunder. One did not have to seek far to determine that the reason for the recommendation was the desire of a high official of the society to pay a political debt.

At this point the reader might well ask, "What do you mean by a graduate of an unapproved school? I thought that such schools went out of existence years ago." The answer is that, although the Flexner report was published in 1910, unapproved schools continued to exist for the next 38 years. The last one was not closed until 1948. And some states continue to license their graduates either legally or illegally. In fact, as recently as 1967, 11 graduates of unapproved schools were licensed by endorsement in ten different states. Therefore, a small number continue to practice in the United States although their ranks are being continually thinned by the natural process of attrition due to death or disability. In the case mentioned above the stigma of politics could be traced all the way back to the original licensure of the individual which was accomplished illegally through political pressure.

35

As boards of medical examiners must fulfill important educational and examining functions, as well as act as disciplinary bodies, one would assume that at least minimal qualifications for membership would be defined. This is not true; in fact the laws of four states do not set forth any requirements at all. In the states which do attempt to prescribe qualifications the most commonly encountered one pertains to period of residence in the state; 23 laws specify that board members must have resided in the state for minimum periods of from three to ten years. The most common period named is five years. In addition, most of the laws require the prospective board member to be a licensed, actively practicing physician. Ten laws merely state that he must be a licensed physician, while in two states he must have an M.D. degree; one provides that the candidate must be a "regularly graduated physician." Only two state laws attempt to spell out personal qualifications; one says that he "must be learned and skilled in medicine, licensed in the state," while another requires him to be "a reputable physician and surgeon."

In only 17 states are educational requirements for board members specifically defined; the definitions are variable and often vague. In five states a board member must be a graduate of a reputable medical school, in four a graduate of a legally chartered school, in four a graduate of an accredited school (which is undefined). In two states the school must be recognized by the state, whatever that means, and in one, the school must be in good standing but with whom is not stated.

Eight state laws contain definite restrictions against a board member belonging to the faculty of a medical school. One goes so far as to prohibit a candidate from having a "vested interest" in any medical school, while another says, "No member shall be a stockholder or a member of the faculty of any medical school." No doubt the latter prohibition is a throwback to the pre-Flexner days of proprietary schools.

From many conversations which I have held with board members, I have concluded that the main reason for forbidding them to belong to the faculties of medical schools is to avoid partiality towards the graduates of any school. Furthermore, as some believe that the most important function of the board of medical examiners is to assess the ability of the candidate for licensure to practice medicine, they think that this can best be done by practicing physicians without academic prejudices of any kind. For example, one state board secretary made the statement, in discussing examination questions, that he could tell from reading the answers to two or three essay type questions whether or not the candidate was fit to practice medicine in his state! One can only marvel at his perspicacity and hope that he does not ignore the other answers. Or possibly his fellow board members waste their time by further reading. In other words, many boards believe that their main function is to judge the fitness of the candidate to practice. And while most members are not as dogmatic as the secretary quoted above, their effectiveness in fulfilling this function is indeed questionable in view of their lack of academic attainments, which I shall consider in detail below.

California obviously does not frown upon members of faculties of medical schools serving on the board of medical examiners. Its law specifies that not more than two of the members of the board shall be full-time members of the faculties of medical schools. One state, Nebraska, takes the opposite view from those who believe that medical educators have no place on boards. The Nebraska law states that two members must be officials or members of the instructional staff of a class A medical school in the state. Obviously the suspicion of educators prevalent in other states is not shared by Nebraska.

California is also unique in its requirement that one member must represent the public. People familiar with medical licensure look askance at the presence of a "layman" on a medical board. They ask, "What can he contribute to the problems of medical licensure?" Or they say, "The nature of medical boards requires that their members possess much technical knowledge." But we must not lose sight of the fact that boards of medical examiners are public bodies whose sole function is to protect the welfare of the public. And how can the interests of the public be better protected than by having a representative on the board? From talking to former members of the California board I have learned that the presence of a non-medical member is not distasteful to them and their original uneasiness caused by the requirement has been allayed.

In many states licensing boards in general have been under fire both from the public and from the legislatures. Many of the boards are accused of existing for the sole purpose of serving the selfish aims of the trades and professions which they represent by excluding outsiders from licensure, thus stifling competition. Furthermore, many boards have been guilty of conducting their deliberations in secrecy and of imparting minimal information to the governor and to the public whom they serve. In some states attempts to remedy these abuses have been made by placing all boards under departments of licensure administered by nonprofessional people. Such regulation is not welcomed by many physicians who believe correctly that this takes away their rightful powers of self-regulation. On the other hand, boards of medical examiners have not always operated properly and their conduct might well be subjected to more careful scrutiny. This could be accomplished by appointing a public member, who admittedly would possess no professional skills; for this reason he should not be allowed to vote on matters purely professional.

No doubt eventually more and more state legislatures will require public representation upon public boards and the physicians will conclude that this is not an unreasonable requirement. However, the governor must exercise great care in his appointment of a public member, bearing in mind that his function is truly to represent the public and not solely to act as a watchdog over imagined nefarious machinations of the professional members.

In the laws of only three states can I find any open reference to political considerations in the appointment of board members. While the language varies, the implication in all three of these laws is that no more than a majority of one can belong to the same political party. The statutes are silent regarding political independents so we can only guess as to whether or not they might be acceptable. We also cannot know whether or not all of the board members always belong to the generally recognized political parties. This stipulation in the law may be good or bad depending upon the viewpoint of the observer. However, it is upsetting to the idealists in the medical profession who believe that boards of medical examiners must be above all political considerations. But some of these same idealists ignore the existence of medical politics to which I have already referred.

Two medical practice laws, those of New Jersey and Michigan, contain surprising anachronisms. In referring to appointment of board members the Michigan statute states that the governor shall appoint them from a list submitted by the medical society with the stipulation "that 1 member of said board shall at all times be a homeopathic physician who is a graduate of a school of medicine known as homeopathic." The New Jersey board, a composite one, is also appointed by the governor from a list submitted by the respective societies. In referring to the medical members the law states that "the said board shall consist of nine graduates of schools of medicine who shall possess the degree of M.D., of whom five shall be old school physicians, three shall be homeopaths, and one an eclectic. . . ." The apparent tenacity of the homeopaths is amazing. But possibly their inclusion in the boards of New Jersey and Michigan is due to lack of recent revisions of the laws of these states. Or are they really still influential?

To learn about the educational backgrounds of individual board members, I studied the biographical sketches in the *American Medical Directory* of all of the 328 M.D.'s listed as members of the Federation of State Medical Boards of the United States. They were scrutinized as to type of medical practice and as to certification by specialty boards. Although at first glance it might appear arbitrary to classify any physician who is not certified by a specialty board as a general practitioner, in reality this is a practical method. While many physicians list themselves as general practitioners, others, possessing little claim to specialized knowledge, list two specialties and, although they might belong to so-called specialty societies these often have little standing and their requirements for membership are not strict. Although I realize I might be taken to task for my insistence upon board certification in defining a specialist, diplomates have at least fulfilled certain minimal educational requirements and have demonstrated knowledge in their specialties by having passed prescribed examinations. On the other hand, many well-trained specialists no doubt, for various reasons, have not bothered to become board certified.

Having defined my terms, I submit that out of 328 physicians listed as members of the Federation of State Medical Boards of the United States, 198 or 60 per cent are general practitioners. The specialties are represented by the following numbers of board members: General Surgery, 35; Internal Medicine, 26; Pathology, 15; Obstetrics and Gynecology, 15; Radiology, 8; Pediatrics, 7; Ophthalmology, 5; Public Health, 4; Urology, 4; Neurosurgery, 3; Orthopedics, 2; Dermatology, 2; one each from Colon and Rectal Surgery, Otolaryngology, Physical Medicine, and Anesthesiology.

There are five boards all of whose members are general practitioners with no claims to specialties. A total of 25 more boards contain a majority of general practitioners, while 16 contain a majority of specialists. Four have equal representation of specialists and general practitioners.

From the preponderance of general practitioners on boards it is obvious that few members are selected because of their special educational attainments. Therefore, all too frequently members are called upon to examine in subjects with which they are not familiar. For example, it is particularly painful for the radiologist who is called upon to examine in obstetrics or the general practitioner who must examine in the fine points of the basic sciences with which he has had little or no contact since he graduated from medical school; little wonder that many of the examination questions are based upon theories long outmoded.

There is a notable lack of balance on the boards as far as specialist members are concerned. It is not uncommon to find two or three members of the same specialty on one board. I found only one well balanced board consisting of a pathologist, a surgeon, an obstetrician and gynecologist, an internist, and a general practitioner. Notably lacking on this board is a psychiatrist but no doubt psychiatric consultation is readily available.

Those who believe in a preponderance of general practitioners on boards of medical examiners present the following argument: The primary function of medical examiners is to determine whether or not candidates for licensure are fit to practice medicine. All boards license physicians to practice medicine and surgery, not a specialty. Ergo, the general practitioner is the best judge of the qualifications of a candidate to engage in general practice. I have even heard one of the most ardent champions of general practice state that membership on boards should be confined to general practitioners, all of whom should reside in small towns. A glance at the membership of this man's board convinced me that he is politically powerful in his state because all of the members are general practitioners and all live in towns ranging in size from small to minute; moreover the state capital, which is the metropolis of the entire region, lacks representation! But, granted that candidates for licensure must possess broad general knowledge to be licensed as "physicians and surgeons," general practice as such is not taught in any medical school. Therefore, while certain general practitioners might have much to contribute to state boards, by no means can they furnish the complete answer to the problems of medical licensure.

Another interesting consideration is the ages of the members of boards of medical examiners. As only four state laws place restrictions upon the number of terms a member may serve, it is understandable that many senior citizens hold on to their positions year after year. The oldest board member in my survey was 82 and two others were over 80. On the other hand the youngest member was 35 and five members under the age of 40 were found. The average age of all of the board members was 58.3 years. The highest average age of an individual board was 65.7 years. The members of five more boards averaged more than 65 years of age. The youngest average age was 44 years and there are three additional boards whose average age was under 50.

Longevity of board members offers advantages and disadvantages. Almost all boards have the dual functions of examining prospective practitioners and enforcing discipline. To carry out the latter, mature judgement and tolerance are prime requisites; perhaps we can assume that these qualities can be attained with age. On the other hand, it is difficult to understand how some of the senior citizens on boards can keep abreast of new developments in medical science and modern techniques of examining. This doubt can be confirmed by inspection of the examinations of several states where the same antiquated questions recur with dreary regularity year after year. Some boards are circumventing this problem by obtaining their questions from outside examination services. But in certain states they are forbidden to do this by attorney generals' rulings that this is an illegal delegation of the authority of the board to an outside agency. Nevertheless, one cannot escape the conclusion that some of the older boards are handicapped by the fact that the advanced ages of the members are not conducive to progress in any field. No doubt the problem of the superannuated public servant will persist in all of the states which place no limit upon the number of terms a member may serve. I am convinced that all members should serve staggered terms to insure continuity of experience. My conviction is strengthened by the administrative chaos which is sometimes caused by the politically motivated governor who makes a clean sweep of members in order that he can fill the board with his own favorites.

The terms of office of board members vary. In the laws of three states it is not specified, in 20 states it is four years, in 10 it is five years. In the other states the terms range from three to eight years. In only four states are there restrictions on reappointment.

From a study of the provisions in the medical practice laws pertaining to financial remuneration of board members, one can only conclude that the majority are selfless public servants who neither expect nor receive financial gain from their positions. As most are actively practicing physicians, weighed down by the demands of their patients, and by their hospital and civic duties, their service upon state boards makes great extra demands upon their time and energies. Many of them are charged with the responsibility of formulating examination questions as well as grading large numbers of examinations of the essay type, the answers to which are often handwritten in exasperatingly illegible fashion. Their patience may also be tried by lengthy hearings drawn out by defense attorneys whose motives are to confuse rather than to search for the truth.

While great variation in the methods of remuneration was found, the majority of laws provide only for nominal per diem payments usually with the addition of expenses. The members are reimbursed only while they are actively engaged in their duties. The per diem fees range from $10.00 to $20.00 although in one state the members are allowed only $6.00, while in two they are paid $50.00. There is usually additional allowance for the secretary who is the administrative officer of the board.

Board members, as do other public servants, often find themselves targets of attack from the public, the press, and even from their professional colleagues. This hazard, added to the many onerous duties which they must perform with minimal financial remuneration, causes one to wonder just why so many of them accept reappointment year after year. In fact many cling tenaciously to their positions and are deeply wounded when they are replaced. Some of the answers to this question can only fall in the realm of speculation. No doubt members enjoy certain political advantages from their memberships on boards. They have a feeling of belonging and that they are on the "inside" of the state government. Many have ready access to the governor with the result that they can advise him on matters other than licensing affairs. Often the governor turns to the board members for advice on pending legislation of importance to the medical profession as well as to the public. Some board members feel flattered by the implication that their positions label them as leaders of their profession.

Fortunately for our democratic form of government there are many public spirited citizens who graciously give of their time and energies by serving on all sorts of boards and commissions, including those of public hospitals and state universities. No doubt many members of boards of medical examiners serve merely because they feel an obligation to engage in public service. Those who serve for long periods should realize that they run the risk of losing their effectiveness not only by superannuation but also by becoming autocrats who brook no disagreement and stubbornly resist change. That some of the newer members of boards are sometimes so poorly qualified that they must undergo long periods of "on the job training" is a fault of the system which permits appointment of members whose political attributes outweigh their professional qualifications.

From the above studies a composite board member emerges. He is a Caucasian man, a little over 58 years of age (only one woman serves on a board, that of New Hampshire); most likely a general practitioner; if not, a general surgeon or an internist. He is a leader in the medical community and well known to the members of his state medical society. He possesses no singular attributes which qualify him to judge the academic attainments of applicants for licensure, but he is sincere in carrying out his duties and may seek help in formulating his examination questions. He is a graduate of an approved American medical school and is better qualified to carry out the disciplinary duties of his office than the educational and examining functions. He does not serve with thought of financial gain. If he remains in office long he must learn to ignore the political pressures which are frequently brought to bear upon him and he must become inured to the assaults of his critics both within and outside the medical profession.

For his public service the board member receives blame more often than praise and, as is the lot of all public servants, he must be prepared to deal with a hostile press. In addition, he is often unfairly attacked by his medical colleagues, not necessarily because of malice but through ignorance of the issues. Allowing for the usual human frailties, one can only conclude that under the best of circumstances the average member of a board of medical examiners is a dedicated public servant.

Bibliography

American Medical Association. 1967. *American Medical Directory.* 24th ed. Chicago.

Federation of State Medical Boards of the United States. 1956. *A Guide to the Essentials of a Modern Medical Practice Act.*

Pearson, H. L. 1963. Political and Economic Barriers to Universal Endorsement and Reciprocity. *Fed. Bull.* 50:256–62.

THE FEDERATION OF STATE
MEDICAL BOARDS OF THE UNITED STATES

For many years, Dr. Walter L. Bierring was so closely identified with the Federation of State Medical Boards that the two were almost synonymous (see *Fed. Bull.* 48: 278–313, Walter L. Bierring Memorial Issue, October, 1961). One of its earliest members, Dr. Bierring became secretary of the Federation and editor of its publication, the *Federation Bulletin*, in August, 1915, and served continuously until 1960. Although he had many other interests, including a term as president of the American Medical Association, Dr. Bierring remained devoted to the Federation throughout his long and distinguished career; he provided the continuity needed for the survival of an organization composed of people and institutions representing a diversity of interests.

Early in his career a near tragedy occurred when his left leg was amputated because of a diagnosis of cancer. Later, although there was reason to doubt the diagnosis, Dr. Bierring was never bitter because of his experience, and never let his handicap dampen his zest for a long life of accomplishment.

This remarkable man was born in Davenport, Iowa, on July 15, 1868, of Danish parents. He received his M.D. degree from the State University of Iowa in 1892. He then spent two years in postgraduate study in Heidelberg, Vienna, and Paris. At the Pasteur Institute he worked with those medical giants of the day, Pasteur, Metchnikoff, and Roux, an experience which he was never to forget.

Returning to the United States, he began the first of what might well be called four careers. He became a teacher at the State University of Iowa where he was professor of pathology and bacteriology for many years. Later he was professor of the theory and practice of medicine at the same school. During a hiatus of three years he was professor of medicine at Drake University. During this period he introduced to the Middle West many of the advances in medicine which he had learned about in Europe.

Dr. Bierring's second career, as a practicing consultant in medicine, began in 1913. In this capacity, for the next 20 years, he was able to apply the fundamental principles of the basic sciences in which he was so well versed, to the practice of medicine. Although known primarily as a clinician during those years, he never lost his interest in medical education.

His third career began in 1933 when Dr. Bierring was appointed health commissioner for the State of Iowa, a post which he held for the next 20 years. From 1953 until his death in 1961 he was director of the Iowa Health Department's division of gerontology, and heart and chronic diseases.

The fourth career of Dr. Bierring was that of medical statesman. Although intertwined with the first three, it must be mentioned because of his many contributions to medicine outside of his scientific fields. Against considerable odds he worked hard to improve interstate reciprocal relations between medical boards in this country. An inveterate traveller, his interest in medical education was not confined to the United States but caused him to range far and wide in other countries. During one of his journeys abroad he arranged reciprocal relations between the National Board of Medical Examiners and the Conjoint and Triple Qualification Boards in Britain.

His unwavering interest in the problems of medical licensure probably began during his seven year term as president of the Iowa State Board of Medical Examiners. He also served on the National Board of Medical Examiners and was its president for four years. His medical statesmanship was also demonstrated by his service to the American Medical Association; for several years he was a member of its House of Delegates and later he was its president. Long after the expiration of his term as president he continued to maintain close contacts with the officers of the Association and was largely responsible for the ties between the AMA's Council on Medical Education and the Federation. By no means unimportant was the generous financial support of the AMA to the Federation which was granted mainly through his efforts through the years.

Well-deserved honors, both in the United States and in other countries, were heaped upon Dr. Bierring during his lifetime. One of these was the AMA Distinguished Service medal. In 1955, while he was still active in the organization, the Federation of State Medical Boards established the annual Walter L. Bierring Lectureship. It was indeed fitting that the Federation did not wait until after his death to institute a memorial lectureship and that he was able to be present at six of these lectures which honored him. Although some of the introductions to the lectures were so flowery as to resemble eulogies for the dead, Dr. Bierring always accepted them with grace and modesty.

Dr. Bierring's mind was clear and active until the end of his life. On his 90th birthday he was immortalized in a cartoon by the late great "Ding" Darling of the *Des Moines Register and Tribune.* He was depicted as offering an hour glass to Father Time and saying, "Fill it up again!" Dr. Bierring died in 1961 at the age of 92.

Throughout his long association with the Federation Dr. Bierring was its guiding spirit and preserved its integrity during several difficult periods including two world wars. His passing left a vacuum in the leadership of the Federation. Although he gave the outward impression of being the quiet diplomat, he showed strength when necessary and ran the Federation with an iron hand in a velvet glove for many years. Fortunately most of his decisions were sound but, in later years particularly, some of the younger members of the Federation became impatient with Dr. Bierring's adherence to the status quo and his reluctance to support changes. But, to his credit, he ran the organization as a gentlemen's club, a quality which is missed today by many of its older members.

The Federation of State Medical Boards of the United States was formed in 1913 by a merger of the National Confederation of State Medical Examining and Licensing Boards and the American Confederation of Reciprocating Examining and Licensing Medical Boards. While the primary aims of the two organizations were different, their union was logical. According to Bierring (1923), the National Confederation of State Medical Examining and Licensing Boards, formed in 1891, was primarily concerned with improving the standards of medical education through the influence of state board regulations and licensure examinations. One of its most important early activities was the appointment of a committee to make a survey of minimum entrance requirements to medical schools. Dr. Bierring said, "Its report in 1899 distinctly influenced the unifying of preliminary education and promoted the general adoption of a full high school training as a requirement for admission to medical schools, which later gradually led to the one and two year premedical college requirement."

Baker (1937) said that the Confederation forced the flagrantly commercial medical schools out of existence and its work resulted in great improvement in medical education. He pointed out that the primary objective of this Confederation was to improve medical education by the eradication of commercial medical colleges, and to raise the standards of the remaining medical institutions. Possibly Baker was overenthusiastic in his claims for accomplishments of the Confederation but certainly the organization recognized the other forces, such as the American Medical Association, which were working for the improvement of medical education and readily cooperated with them.

In the last years of the 19th century some boards of medical examiners realized that many of the candidates seeking medical licenses were grossly ignorant. Some had never attended medical schools, while many had taken only a few courses in medicine. For licensing, the candidates were only required to pass examinations. Many well trained physicians did not think that this was sufficient; they thought that the boards ought to insist that candidates for licensure should possess medical diplomas. They also believed that those already licensed should not be expected to pass examinations if they wished to move from one state to another. In 1901 a movement was begun to establish a national medical examining board, the certificate of which would allow the holder the right to practice anywhere in the country. The American Medical Association espoused this cause but, after investigation, determined that legislation to provide for it had been delegated to the states by the federal constitution and therefore it was not feasible.

Later, certain prominent members of the medical profession began to advocate plans for a voluntary national examining board. This was submitted to the National Confederation of State Medical Examining and Licensing Boards which disapproved of it. Meanwhile, members of state examining boards became restless over the lack of interstate reciprocity. In 1901 Dr. H. M. Ludwig, secretary of the Wisconsin State Board of Medical Examiners, worked out a plan for reciprocal exchange of physicians with his neighbor, Dr. B. D. Harison, secretary of the Michigan Board. Out of this came the idea for extending the plan to all states and on January 17, 1902 a meeting was called in Chicago which was attended by representatives from Illinois, Indiana, Michigan, and Wisconsin. Thus, the Confederation of Reciprocating State Medical Examining Boards was conceived. Later its membership was increased and its aims broadened to include efforts to improve educational standards and to promote uniform legislation for medical licensure.

By 1910 the president of the American Confederation of Reciprocating Medical Examining and Licensing Medical Boards stated his belief that the primary purpose for which the organization had been formed had been fulfilled. This facilitated negotiations with the National Confederation for merger. It was accomplished under the interested and watchful eyes of representatives of the Association of American Medical Colleges, the Council on Medical Education of the American Medical Association, and the Carnegie Foundation for the Advancement of Teaching. Dr. Arthur Dean Bevan declared that it was desirable that there should be in this country one strong organization of state examining and licensing boards and with little difficulty the merger was arranged; the name chosen for the new organization was The National Federation of State Medical Boards. On February 28, 1912, when the constitution and by-laws were approved, the name was changed to The Federation of State Medical Boards of the United States. The first president of the new organization was Dr. Arthur B. Brown of Louisiana.

The formation of the Federation of State Medical Boards of the United States was well received by the public press. Said *Harper's Weekly* of July 26, 1913, "There should be a hearty welcome from the entire public to the newly formed Federation of State Medical Boards. It not merely aims at an end indisputably desirable, but it seems a feasible and practical plan to accomplish that end." The *New York Times* of July 14, 1913, said, "Recognition of the fact that the treatment of disease is a public rather than a private concern is becoming steadily clearer, day by day, and the Federation's privilege will be to emphasize and extend this truth."

The official publication of the newly formed Federation was the *Federation Quarterly*. But at the third annual meeting in February 1915 the members decided to publish a monthly journal to be known as the *Federation Bulletin*, which has appeared continuously since. Volume 1, Number 1, of the *Federation Bulletin* appeared in April 1915. It was devoted almost entirely to a discussion of uniform licensing laws. Dr. Walter Bierring became secretary of the Federation and editor of the *Bulletin* in August 1915, and was not to relinquish his post until 1960. Since then there have been four editors, the longest term being six years.

The first meeting of the Federation of State Medical Boards of the United States was held in Chicago on February 25, 1913. Topics of discussion on the first program were the following: "Should Medical Boards Require One or More Years of Pre-medical College Work?"; "Should an Internship Be Required?"; "Rules and Regulations Governing Examinations"; "Universal Reciprocity"; "The Methods of State Board Record Keeping"; "The Qualifications of Examiners"; "What Fee Should Be Charged for Examination?"

The roster of members included 28 state medical boards, Arkansas being represented twice—by the Arkansas State

Eclectic Medical Board of Examiners and by the State Medical Board of the Arkansas Medical Society. But apparently the dual representation of Arkansas was soon discontinued, for Dr. Bierring (1915), in his first editorial, stated that 27 state boards belonged to the Federation, representing more than three-fourths of the population of the United States. He also said, "If the state boards do not wake up and meet present day conditions and criticisms, it will not be long before some sort of a federal board will replace them." It is interesting that we continue to hear the same predictions today, albeit they are expressed with a greater sense of urgency because of the increasing involvement of the federal government in all medical affairs.

The purpose of the Federation is stated in its original constitution: "The object shall be to develop and maintain reasonably high and uniform standards of medical licensure in the United States. Contributing toward this end the Federation shall endeavor (a) to obtain accurate knowledge of the standards of preliminary and of medical education; the rules adopted and methods employed by the medical boards of the various states of this country and of other countries; (b) to publish a bulletin by which this information may be disseminated among its members; and (c) to further interstate endorsement of medical licensure."

Perusal of early volumes of the *Federation Bulletin* reveals preoccupation of the Federation with the problems posed by the prevalence of quacks; but also early in its history the organization was interested in educational standards and quality of state board examinations (see Baldy, 1916). Baldy, president of the Pennsylvania Board in 1916, took issue with the policy of the boards of medical examiners of asking detailed questions on the fundamental facts of medicine. Prophetically he said he was a strong believer that the state, in its licensing examinations, should not examine in the fundamental sciences directly; it should confine its tests to practical questions, or questions of practice, questions that the applicant could not answer, however, unless he understood the general principles and the main facts of the fundamental sciences. Obviously Baldy's ideas anticipated by many years the philosophy of the Examination Institutes Committee of the Federation.

Since its founding the Federation has labored under several handicaps. First, it has never had any legal authority so that its only function has been to advise the member state boards and to attempt to correlate their activities. Therefore, many well-meaning resolutions have come to naught and have been ignored by the boards. Second, because of its national scope it has been a diffuse organization with officers and members of its governing body widely scattered over the United States. There has never been more than one annual meeting of the entire membership, and interim meetings of the executive committee have not been held more than twice a year; recently the meetings have been reduced to one a year. Consequently, changes come about at a snail's pace and sound proposals which have been assigned for further study to committees often have either been forgotten or adopted only after long delays.

But, thanks to Dr. Bierring and a few of his more enlightened followers who have arranged the annual programs, some of the pressing problems of the day were at least recognized and discussed even though they were not solved. For example, the 1916 program of the Federation was devoted entirely to a symposium on the National Board of Medical Examiners. Among the participants were Dr. Arthur Dean Bevan and Surgeon General William Crawford Gorgas. After a detailed presentation of the aims and standards of the National Board, the members of the Federation were invited to express their opinions. The early members of the Federation were highly vocal, as are today's members, and a total of 16 of them spoke for or against the National Board and its proposed relationship to the state boards. In view of some of the recent attacks on the National Board by a Federation member from Texas, it is interesting that this state was represented by three members in the original discussion. One, Dr. C. E. Cantrell of Greenville, expressed bitter opposition to the National Board and erroneously announced that a request for approval by the House of Delegates of the American Medical Association had been tabled. Dr. Cantrell was called to account for his error but he remained adamant in his opposition. Dr. T. J. Crowe of Dallas also took a dim view of the National Board, darkly hinting that it was a step towards federal control of licensure; this, despite the repeated protestations of the founders of the National Board that it only sought to be a voluntary qualifying body. In 1968 attacks upon the National Board continued despite the fact that it has never attempted to become a national licensing agency.

Another example of the awareness of the early members of the Federation of the problems of the day is emphasized in an editorial by Dr. Bierring in 1917. He recognized the dislocations of medical practices which were bound to result from World War I. He warned the state boards that, because of the exigencies of war, they must arrange for flexibility in their laws and regulations concerning the early graduation of physicians before completion of the usual four-year medical curriculum. He thought that such early graduation should not count against them in licensing and he even advocated that they be given credit for military training in the medical corps.

During Dr. Bierring's long term as secretary of the Federation its meetings were always closely integrated with those of the Congress on Medical Education of the American Medical Association. On several occasions the Federation held jointly sponsored sessions with the Council, with the Association of American Medical Colleges, or with both of these agencies. But after his death, Dr. Bierring's influence rapidly waned. The ties between the Federation and the Council on Medical Education became looser, and at one point relations became strained. The Federation seemed to be floundering in several directions at once. Frequently, in response to the demands of an anti-intellectual segment of the organization which became influential out of all proportion to its importance, the Federation's programs were in direct conflict with those of the Council. These members shunned discussion of problems of medical education and openly stated that they could find nothing which interested them in the programs of the Council. They were interested only in licensure and not in education— as if the two could be dissociated! At any rate they soon found themselves in direct conflict with several of the members of the Federation who were interested in the broader aspects of education and licensure.

That the same old problems have arisen year after year can be seen in the past programs of the Federation and in many of the articles which have appeared in the *Federation Bulletin*. I have already noted that one of the topics on the first program in 1913 was "Universal Reciprocity." Since then this subject has been discussed formally on 18 additional programs, not to mention the endless wrangles over the problem which have been heard in the informal meetings of the executive officers of the state boards. As recently as 1968 another paper on the subject was presented and it contributed nothing new.

Another recurring subject is the question of the basic science laws. This topic has appeared on the annual programs 14 times with no sign of agreement. Many members of the Federation have long considered basic science laws to be useless anachronisms; but to date only four states have repealed their laws. These actions were taken without the help of the Federation, which refused to take a stand either for or against these laws.

The problem of the graduates of foreign medical schools has also received its share of discussion, having been included in the programs 18 times. But recently, although the problem is far from solution, it has been discussed less frequently partly because of the efficient functioning of the Educational Council for Foreign Medical Graduates which is described in another chapter.

Disciplinary problems have been discussed at 14 meetings and no doubt this will be a recurring topic for many years to come. These problems can never be completely solved and the recurring discussions indicate a healthy attitude on the part of the boards in their desire to perform one of their most important duties efficiently.

Frequently new and fresh ideas are presented on the programs. For example, as recently as 1967 a whole morning was devoted to a panel discussion on the subject, "Are There State Licensure Barriers To Innovations in Medical Education?"

This problem had been discussed four times previously, the first time in 1923. I call attention to this, not to label it as an exercise in futility, but to stress the fact that medical practice laws should be re-examined periodically to determine whether or not they are impeding progress in medical education.

Much oratory and time have been wasted on the question of the Federation's writing a model medical practice act. I find this topic recurred five times in the Federation programs. Finally in 1956 the organization was able to agree on a compromise document called, "A Guide to the Essentials of a Model Medical Practice Act." (See Appendix.)

The Federation of State Medical Boards of the United States should be a truly national organization with a broad view of all of the problems of state licensure. Its failure to attain stature is due in large part to the dearth of people with vision among its leaders and the provincial viewpoint of many of its members. In listening to its deliberations, one is reminded of some of the debates carried on in state legislatures in which the viewpoint of each participant is limited by the boundaries of his particular county. Thus, many of the members of the Federation can see only the problems of their own states, most of which they think they have solved; and they are anxious to inform the members of their solutions and how they do things at home. They forget that medical education and science are not regional, that principles of medical ethics and discipline are not based upon local custom, and that unprofessional conduct is the same in California as in Maine.

Although much of the impotence of the Federation is due to its lack of legal authority and the diffuseness of the organization, it still has the potential to become a force for good both in medical licensure and education. The most significant forward step is represented by the Federation Licensing Examination which is described elsewhere. At the end of the first year of operation seven states had used it in examining some 900 candidates for licensure. New York and California have now agreed to use it so that in 1969 the number of candidates should be double that in 1968. In addition at least seven other states have indicated their desire to adopt the examinations as soon as legal and administrative obstacles can be overcome. If used properly the Federation Licensing Examination could establish uniformly high medical licensing standards throughout the United States for the first time. But a serious drawback is that the states can use the examinations as they choose and already two boards have decided that the failure rates were too high for political comfort and have revised the examination scores upward. Although the Federation is powerless to prevent this, the true scores of the candidates are filed with the Federation and these can be obtained by the officials of any state board.

If the practice of grading upward the scores of the Federation Licensing Examination spreads, the purpose of the entire project will be defeated and the licensing situation will never rise out of the slough of multiple standards and special favors in which it has floundered for so many years.

For many years the Federation has had a standing legislative advisory committee which has never been active. This is partly due to members' reluctance to advise the boards, apparently because of their fear of offending the supporters of states' rights, and also to the seeming apathy and lack of imagination of members of the committee. The Federation could also be of value in advising boards and medical societies in the revisions of their medical practice acts. Although the Federation published its "Guide to the Essentials of a Modern Medical Practice Act" in 1956, few states have used it. And this is not due to lack of soundness of the document, which has been much more freely quoted by lawyers than by physicians.

To become a real force for good the Federation must have strong and imaginative leadership which it now appears to lack. The president serves for only one year, so that no matter how vigorous his administration or how good his ideas, he is able to carry out few if any of them during his brief term of office. Whenever he proposes changes he is usually blocked by the champions of the status quo. Moreover, the constitution of the Federation does not require the president and the other officers to be active members of their boards of medical examiners, so that frequently the leadership is provided by a succession of "lame ducks" who, although they may have been active in the past, may be far removed from the everyday problems of licensure by the time they assume office.

The financial support of the Federation comes from two main sources: the dues of the member state boards and a grant from the American Medical Association which has been renewed annually since 1963. The grant from the American Medical Association was originally requested for the purpose of establishing a central office, something the Federation had never had before. In addition to providing continuity of administration, the central office was supposed to act as a clearing house for all information regarding medical licensure and disciplinary actions. To date it has made few contributions in either field. Whatever information the central office has been able to gather concerning licensure can easily be found in the annual State Board Number of the *Journal of the American Medical Association*, and the files of the Department of Investigation of the American Medical Association provide information regarding disciplinary actions far more complete than do the partially duplicating records of the Federation. The Federation Licensing Examination is financially self-supporting.

The Federation is involved in varying degrees with several other organizations. It has five representatives on the National Board of Medical Examiners. At present two of its members serve on the Executive Committee, the interim governing and policy making body of the Board. From public statements which have been made at meetings of the Federation one can only conclude that there is sharp division of opinion regarding acceptance of the National Board. Obviously some of the Federation representatives on the National Board believe that they have been appointed to serve as watchdogs to report on the activities of this outstanding body.

A positive contribution has been made by the Federation toward solving the problems of the graduates of foreign medical schools. The Federation was active in the organization of the Educational Council for Foreign Medical Graduates and the present president of the Council, Dr. Joseph Combs, is a representative of the Federation. The functions of the Council are discussed elsewhere in this book.

The Federation is also represented on the Internship Review Committee of the Council on Medical Education of the American Medical Association. For several years, through its representative, Dr. C. J. Glaspell, the Federation contributed to postgraduate medical education, and one hopes that his good work will be carried on by his successors.

Another important field in which the Federation should be active is the Advisory Board for the Medical Specialties. The Federation is entitled to two members on this board but the representatives frequently have attended meetings irregularly if at all. I regret this, because the Advisory Board is assuming increasing importance and affords the Federation an opportunity to make positive contributions to medicine.

More than one disillusioned member of the Federation has privately called it an impotent debating society. But, to be fair, I must point to a few real contributions of the organization. Its chief value is the opportunity it affords the members of the state boards to meet each other and to exchange information and ideas. This is particularly advantageous to the secretaries and other executive officers. They can become personally acquainted with their counterparts in other states, which certainly facilitates communication. This has been accomplished in spite of the fact that most of the annual meetings of the executive officers of the boards have turned out to be quarrelsome affairs due to lack of organization.

Certainly the Federation's part in attempting to solve the foreign graduate problem has been useful, as mentioned above.

The annual programs of the Federation in the past have more often than not proven interesting to its members, but, again, this varies from year to year depending on the leadership.

The Federation of State Medical Boards of the United States has the potential of becoming an important influence in medical licensure, discipline, and education; but, in the 55 years of its existence, it has never found its rightful place. Undoubtedly many of its more aggressive members would like to see it assume a more influential position; but there is internal disagreement as to its proper objectives and their mode of development. While I do not advocate a return to the past, perhaps the Federation should concentrate on the few fields in which it has been effective and abandon the dreams of glory of some of its members. Its effectiveness is negated by the diffuseness of the members, their reluctance voluntarily to surrender any of their states' rights, and their suspicion of the sincere efforts of anyone to standardize licensure throughout the United States on a high level.

Bibliography

Baker, J. N. 1937. The Federation: Its Origin, History and Obligations. *Fed. Bull.* 23:72–90.
Baldy, J. M. 1916. Examinations For Licensure To Practice Medicine. *Fed. Bull.* 2:126–27.
Bierring, W. L. 1915. Time to Go Ahead. *Fed. Bull.* 1:49–50.
———. 1923. The First Decade of Federation Activities. *Fed. Bull.* 9:58–69.
———. 1956. Medical Licensure After Forty Years. *Fed. Bull.* 43:101–13.

CHAPTER FIVE

THE NATIONAL BOARD
OF MEDICAL EXAMINERS

No account of medical licensure would be complete without inclusion of a discussion of the history, aims, and methods of the National Board of Medical Examiners. While it has never had any legal standing as a licensing body, it has exerted a profound influence over medical standards for many years. The Board's main objective was defined in its original constitution, namely, "To prepare and administer qualifying examinations of such high quality that legal agencies governing the practice of medicine in each state may, at their discretion, grant successful candidates a license without further examination." To understand completely the reason for the founding of the National Board, one must consider the state of medical licensing procedures early in the twentieth century.

At the beginning of the twentieth century, although the majority of the states had established medical licensing boards, they had not solved the problem of interstate reciprocity and endorsement. Only a few state boards would recognize the credentials of others. In addition to provincialism and jealous guarding of states' rights, the lack of uniformity of standards acted as a barrier then, as today. According to Womack (1965)* some examining boards scrutinized a candidate with unusual care, while others did not. Political influences were also at work and they only served to lower standards in some states so that they could not maintain the respect of other boards.

* I have drawn freely upon Dr. Womack's article in the entire account of the history and development of the National Board of Medical Examiners.

In 1902 an editorial appeared in the *Journal of the American Medical Association* which called attention to the need of devising some method for overcoming the anomalous conditions regarding the regulation of the practice of medicine in the various states. Prophetically, the editorial said, ". . . but reciprocity will never be universal among all the states, at least until there is much more uniformity in legislation than now prevails or that is likely to prevail for some years. But even a uniformity of laws will not suffice; there must be some uniformity in tests and standards, which will never come because of the multiplicity of boards of medical examiners, the majority of which are created by political influence and not by the selection of men qualified for the positions of examiners in scientific medicine" (AMA, 1902). The suggested solution to the problem was the establishment of a national board of medical examiners to examine physicians for qualification for positions in the federal government. The editorial proposed that the board be appointed by the President of the United States and that the preliminary education of candidates and the examinations would be of such high quality that eventually the state boards would be willing to recognize a certificate from this board.

At a meeting of the Committee on National Legislation of the American Medical Association held in 1902 the subject of interstate reciprocity was discussed. Representatives of all of the states attending the meeting recommended that a plan for the formation of a voluntary national board of medical examiners be submitted to the House of Delegates. This was opposed by the National Confederation of Medical Examining and Licensing Boards of the United States, one of the parent organizations of the Federation of State Medical Boards. The House of Delegates appointed a committee to consider the question but no action resulted.

Problems concerning interstate reciprocity continued to increase and the state boards could not or would not solve them. Again the idea of a national board as a solution was discussed in the *Journal of the American Medical Association*, this time in a letter to the editor by Dr. John M. Dodson, Dean of

Rush Medical College (Dodson, 1906). He pointed to the inability of the state boards to agree on minimal standards for licensure and the need for an outside, impartial agency to set standards. He suggested that the state boards voluntarily accept the examinations of this agency and said that the survival of a national board would depend upon its excellence. Specifically he suggested the use of experts to formulate questions for the examinations. Said Dodson, "We must come to recognize in this country, as they do abroad, that the business of examining is one demanding special training and experience, particularly in teaching, and that examinations can not be satisfactorily made by the average general practitioners who constitute the personnel for the several state boards." No action came from this.

In 1914 another editorial appeared proposing a national board (AMA, 1914). The following year, Dr. W. L. Rodman presented the subject again to the American Medical Association when he devoted the major part of his presidential address to a discussion of the national board. He discussed in detail the problems caused by multiple licensing boards with no uniform standards of excellence; he then announced that a national board of medical examiners had been formed the previous month with standards similar to those previously recommended by the Council on Medical Education of the American Medical Association. In June 1916 the House of Delegates accepted the report of the Council endorsing the board. "And so," wrote Womack (1965), "was born the National Board of Medical Examiners."

The membership of the original board was indeed distinguished. Representing the United States Navy were Commander E. P. Stitt and Rear Admiral William C. Braisted. From the Army were Col. Louis A. LaGarde and Surgeon General William C. Gorgas. Surgeon General Rupert Blue and his assistant, Dr. W. C. Rucker, represented the United States Public Health Service. From the Federation of State Medical Boards came Dr. Herbert Horlen, while the Association of American Medical Colleges appointed Dr. Isadore Dyer, the American College of Surgeons selected Dr. E. Wyllys Andrews.

Dr. Louis B. Wilson of the Mayo Foundation for Medical Education and Research furnished the prestige of postgraduate medical education. Drs. Victor C. Vaughn and William L. Rodman were the choices of the American Medical Association, while the members at large were Drs. Horace D. Arnold, Austin Flint, and Henry Sewell.

The first states to endorse the certificate of the National Board were Colorado, Idaho, Kentucky, Maryland, New Hampshire, North Carolina, North Dakota, and Vermont.

At the death of Dr. William L. Rodman in 1916, Dr. J. Stewart Rodman, his son and assistant secretary, was named secretary, and Dr. Walter Bierring was elected to serve his unexpired term on the board. Both of these men rendered distinguished service to the Board for many years.

The National Board gave its first examinations October 16–21, 1916 in Washington, D.C. Out of 16 qualified applicants, ten took the examination and five passed. Between 1916 and 1921, examinations were given to 325 qualified applicants, 269 of whom passed.

In 1921, with the help of a grant from the Carnegie Foundation for the Advancement of Teaching, the National Board began to expand its program. At the same time Everett S. Elwood became managing director, a post which he held until 1950. During this period the high quality of the Board's examinations led to acceptance of its certificate for licensure by all but five states.

In 1922 the National Board was incorporated under the laws of the District of Columbia. Its constitution was revised to increase the membership to 21, six representing the federal services, three to be nominated by the Federation of State Medical Boards, and 12 to be elected at large. At present the board membership is still broader and includes five representatives from the federal services, five from the Federation of State Medical Boards, two from the American Medical Association, three from the Association of American Medical Colleges, two from the American Hospital Association, the chairman of each subject test committee, and an indefinite number of members at large.

During the early days of the National Board the examinations involved mainly oral discussions of practical situations and demonstrations of patients. In 1922, Dr. Stewart Rodman presented a new type of examination consisting of three parts: Part I was a written examination on the basic science subjects, Part II, a written examination in the clinical subjects covered in the junior and senior years of medical school, and Part III, a practical examination on clinical and laboratory problems given at the bedside.

According to Womack (1965), "This move in changing the examination form was well thought out, and the new form undoubtedly represented the finest and most discriminating examination for medical proficiency available at the time. The National Board of Medical Examiners quickly began to represent a particular standard of excellence. . . . The Board found its examinations in growing demand as the young American physicians noted what the Board stood for. State boards also found acceptance of the credentials of the National Board more comfortable."

By June 1940, the 25th anniversary of the National Board, some 1200 candidates a year were taking the examination; these represented about 25 per cent of the American medical school graduates.

Meanwhile, the methods and policies of the National Board changed little until after World War II when Dr. John P. Hubbard joined it, first as part-time assistant secretary, later as full-time executive director. Dr. Hubbard brought a full knowledge of objective examinations and statistical methods to the Board. In 1951 and 1952, with the help of the Educational Testing Service, objective examinations were tried in medicine and surgery. These were so successful that a similar form was adopted for all of the subjects of Parts I and II.

The change of format of the examination questions from the essay to the objective type indeed marked an entirely new concept in the preparation and administration of medical examinations. For each subject a committee of outstanding teachers in their respective fields is employed. The members construct subject items, send them to each other for criticism, and then meet at the office of the National Board for one or two days for final construction of the examinations. After the examinations have been given they meet again, criticize the results, and try to improve the next examination.

Recently the National Board made radical changes in Part III (Hubbard, 1968). Before 1961 this part was conducted at the bedside. For several reasons, including variability of the examination in different centers because of the inconsistencies of the individual examiners as well as the patients presented, the Board began to seek ways of improving it. First it was necessary to arrive at a definition of clinical competence. This was carried out by the "critical incident" technique. According to Hubbard and his colleagues on the staff of the board (Hubbard, Levit, Schumacher, Schnabel, 1965), physicians and residents, all of whom had direct responsibility for the supervision of interns, were asked by means of interviews and questionnaires to record clinical situations (incidents) in which they had observed interns doing something that impressed them as good clinical practice or as poor practice. They collected a total of 3,300 incidents from 600 physicians; these were divided equally between good and poor practice. Incidents fell into nine major areas of performance: history, physical examination, tests and procedures, diagnostic acumen, treatment, judgment and skill in implementing care, continuing care, physician-patient relations, and responsibilities as a physician. These incidents gave an answer as to what to test. Three main methods of testing in Part III were adopted. The Board makes motion picture films of patients who exemplify certain clinical manifestations. These are shown to the candidates; at the end of each sequence the film is turned off and the examinees are required to answer a series of multiple choice questions on what they have seen. This is not only a test of diagnostic acumen but also gives the candidates a chance to demonstrate their powers of observation.

The second method used in Part III is known as programmed testing. According to Hubbard (1965), this designation is used because of similarity in principle to programmed teaching—"a step by step progression to carefully defined objectives, each step accompanied by an increment of information essential to the sequential unfolding of the problem." The present mechanics of this part of the examination involve the outline of a clinical situation followed by the presentation of a number of procedures that can be carried out in the management of the patient. Answers to questions concerning additional physical findings, as well as results of X rays and laboratory tests, can be found by erasing certain lines. Thus the candidate obtains information pointing to the next step. If he performs tests which are useless he receives no credit; on the other hand, if he recommends procedures which may be harmful to the patient he is penalized. If he is too careless in his recommendations he might be confronted by a statement such as, "The patient died. Exercise over." This is an excellent test of the ability of a candidate to handle a clinical situation in orderly sequence.

The third method used in Part III is testing of clinical competence by presentation of photographs, charts, reproductions of roentgenograms and photomicrographs; multiple choice questions are asked about these.

On the whole, the new Part III examination has proven satisfactory both to the National Board and to the candidates. Of the motion pictures Levit (1968) said, "We have found that the use of motion pictures has added new dimensions to an objective and reliable test of the physician's skill and judgement in one of the most subtle aspects of the physical examination: the visual evaluation of the patient."

At first some of the state boards of medical examiners were suspicious of the objective type of examinations and ceased to recognize the certificate of the National Board. This is evidenced by the fact that in 1949 all but three states accepted the certificate (AMA, 1950), while in 1953, after the institution of the new system, ten states refused to accept it (AMA, 1959). But gradually the suspicions of the state boards have been allayed as they have noted the extensive studies which have been undertaken to determine the validity and reliability of the method.

Throughout the existence of the National Board the number of state boards accepting its certificate has varied. In 1926 there were 16 states which withheld recognition; by 1936 this number had been reduced to five. During the next decade the number varied from four to six. After the severe setback to the recognition of the Board in 1953, many of the hostile boards were won over so that at present (AMA, 1968) the certificate is accepted as an adequate qualification for licensure by the authorities of the District of Columbia, Puerto Rico, and all of the states except Arkansas, Florida, Georgia, and Kansas. Conditional recognition only is granted by Delaware, Indiana, Louisiana, North Carolina, and Texas. These states accept the certificate only if the diplomate has been licensed in some other state. Some of these states go so far as to require the candidate to have practiced for a year in another state before they will accept his National Board certificate. California requires an oral examination when the application is based upon a certificate issued five or more years before filing. Rhode Island and Wyoming demand practical clinical examinations of diplomates. Georgia will only accept diplomates who were examined in the earlier days of essay type examinations. (Hubbard [1965] observes that this is a curious phenomenon in view of the alleged superiority of objective examinations and the extensive studies that have been carried out which prove their advantages over the essay type.)

Despite the restrictions placed upon recognition of its diplomates, the influence of National Board continues to grow as evidenced by the fact that in 1967, 6,756 licenses were granted on the basis of National Board certificates compared with 4,730 during 1963, 2,900 in 1953 and 700 in 1940.

The District of Columbia and 20 states have separate boards of examiners in the basic sciences and their laws require all candidates for licensure to obtain basic science certificates before they can be considered for medical licensure. The laws of 16 of these states are sufficiently broad to permit them to accept Part I of the National Board in lieu of their own certificates. However, candidates for basic science certificates can be certain of one thing; six states—Colorado, Florida, Michigan,

Nevada, South Dakota, and Texas—will not accept the National Board certificate under any circumstances.

During the past few years the activities of the National Board have been broadened. Several state boards which examine large numbers of candidates have turned to the National Board for questions for their own examinations. Although these are drawn from the pool of National Board questions, they are given as true state board examinations with the imprint of the state on the examination booklets. The examinations are graded by the National Board, the raw scores returned to the states which then determine their own level of passing. In 1967, 16 state boards used questions furnished by the National Board (Hubbard, 1968).

The National Board of Medical Examiners has recently become active in fields not strictly confined to medical licensure. As the resources of the Board have grown, respect for its examinations has increased. The Board has been asked for help in the evaluation of several educational programs. For example, in 1964 the University of Rochester changed its curriculum. In an effort to assess the effects of this change it turned to the National Board which furnished a shortened version of Parts I and II; this has been called a "minitest" (Jason, 1965). In 1967, 15 additional medical schools used this test.

The Air Force and the Army, in an effort to improve their teaching programs, are now using Part III examinations to evaluate their internships (Crouch and Hughes, 1965). These are given at first to test interns before admission to the programs and also at the end of the service to gauge their performance.

The American Board of Neurological Surgery, in 1962, concerned because of the consistently high failure rate of candidates for certification, requested the National Board to develop a one-day test in various basic and clinical subjects related to training in neurosurgery (Hubbard, Furlow, and Matson, 1967). This was designed as a test both of the participants in educational programs and as a measure of the adequacy of the programs themselves.

Projects begun in 1967 included a new examination for the Federation of State Medical Boards of the United States which is described in another chapter; qualifying examinations for the Medical Council of Canada; and cooperation with the American College of Physicians in its medical knowledge self-assessment program.

For many years an increasing number of medical schools have been using the National Board examinations, not necessarily for certification of students, but for outside evaluation of their teaching programs and of their students. During 1967, 54 schools in the United States and Canada required their students to take the examinations of Parts I and II. In an additional 15 schools more than three-quarters of the students took the examinations on a voluntary basis.

Since its inception in 1957 the Educational Council for Foreign Medical Graduates has used selected questions furnished by the National Board in examining graduates of medical schools outside the United States and Canada.

A new and important activity of the National Board is the augmentation of its research program. In the planning stage for a long time, it can now reach fruition with grants totalling $500,000 from the Carnegie Corporation and the Commonwealth Fund. These encompass a three-year period and will be supervised by a Research Advisory Committee headed by Dr. Jack D. Myers, Chairman of the Department of Medicine at the University of Pittsburgh. The main areas of research will be in the core content of the medical school curriculum in relation to the core content of the National Board examinations and the further validation and improvement of measures of testing clinical competence.

Meanwhile, the members of the staff of the National Board of Medical Examiners have not been idle and have made many inquiries both into methods of examination and assessment of their value. In 1952 Cowles and Hubbard made a comparative study of essay and objective examinations. They found that objective test scores corresponded more closely with the evaluation of students in internal medicine and pharmacology by their instructors than did the essay test grades. They claimed that the main advantages of carefully prepared objective examinations were that they offered more reliable evaluation of the students' knowledge and that they lent themselves to statistical analysis by means of which they could be accurately assessed; thus examinations could be improved by suitable revisions.

The National Board has also carefully studied the validity and reliability of objective tests (Cowles and Hubbard, 1954). It has concluded that the tests are valid because of the direct participation of leading medical educators in their construction and the significant correlation of test scores with performance of the student in medical school. It also found that the reliability of the tests was high due mainly to the use of large numbers of questions on each test.

The members of the staff of the National Board have not failed to use the mass of data available from the tests as applied to other fields. For example, Levit, Schumacher and Hubbard (1963) carried out a comparative study of university affiliated and nonaffiliated hospitals in regard to the calibre of interns obtained and of their later competence using the grades of the Part II and Part III examinations. Their conclusions: the affiliated hospitals obtained higher calibre interns but the output was not affected by affiliation if allowance is made for original difference.

Hubbard (1961) has examined the often asked question, "Should physicians be licensed solely on the basis of the M.D. degree from an accredited school?" In studying the scores of graduates of 30 different medical schools on National Board examinations he found wide variation from 36 per cent honors and no failures in one school to 1.5 per cent honors and 31 per cent failures in another. Obviously all accredited schools are not equal.

The National Board has been acutely conscious of the many changes which are occurring in the curricula of medical schools in the United States. It is aware of the fact that its policies must be flexible so that there can be no questions about the Board dictating the educational policies of the schools. Up to 1968 the Board allowed students to take Part I examinations only after the completion of the second year of medical school, Part II after the fourth year, and Part III after the internship. In 1968 the Board made an important change in policy (National Board of Medical Examiners, 1968). Beginning in 1969 the Part I examination questions have been constructed and selected by the six traditional test committees (anatomy, biochemistry, microbiology, pathology, pharmacology, physiology) and by a seventh committee which constructs items in less traditional areas such as genetics and cell biology. All committees are encouraged to broaden the scope of assignments and construct questions which may cross boundaries of disciplines. The examination is presented in a form in which the committee origins of questions is not identified. This interdisciplinary Part I examination is scored as a whole and any candidate who fails is required to repeat the whole examination. However, grades on the traditional subjects are extracted and reported to students, medical schools, and state boards of medical examiners.

The National Board, with its interdisciplinary approach, recognizes the present trend in medical education towards early specialization and increasing use of elective subjects. Therefore a student whose primary interest is in one subject such as surgery, will not be too severely penalized if he is not well versed in the fine points of obstetrics or psychiatry, as he will be judged on his broad grasp of medicine, his strength in one field balancing his weakness in another.

Beginning in 1969 students may, for certification purposes, be admitted to an official regularly scheduled Part I or Part II examination during any year of medical school without restriction due to lack of completion of specified courses or chronological periods of study.

Lest anyone think that the National Board believes that examinations are the answer to all problems, some remarks of Hubbard and Clemens (1960) bring the whole problem into proper perspective. In commenting upon the correlation between faculty ranking of students and ranking by Part II of the National Board examinations, they said, in part, "Nor do we consider it fair or proper to judge medical schools and their teaching solely on the basis of examination results. Any examination is a limited and incomplete evaluation of a student. No matter how good a test may be thought to be, no matter how great a degree of statistical significance is attached to its validity, it is an index of only certain characteristics, measured at one point in time and influenced by variable factors."

From close association with the National Board of Medical Examiners and careful study of its methods, personnel, and objectives over a period of many years, I have become convinced that the quality of its examinations cannot be matched by those of any state board. Yet, there are still four states which will not accept its certificate under any circumstances and an additional ten which grant conditional recognition only. Three of the four states which refuse to accept the certificate of the National Board do so because there is no provision for this in their statutes. Apparently they do not feel inclined to modify them by legislative action. The fourth state does not accept the certificate because of a board regulation; this could be changed at any time. In the 10 states granting limited recognition, this restriction is imposed by board regulations rather than by statute. The reason for this is understandable in such a state as California which reserves the right to give an oral examination to any candidate who finished his training more than five years previously; this is a reasonable safeguard to assure the state board that the candidate has kept himself abreast of advances in medicine. The limitations in some other states are not so easy to understand.

In my many conversations with members of state boards I have never heard any question of the quality of the examinations of the National Board despite the objections of some to the multiple choice format. Therefore, one can be certain that non-recognition is not based upon a question of quality.

Then why do these states refuse to accept the National Board certificate? The answers are not simple, but the most obvious one is that some states are still afraid that by recognizing the National Board they will surrender some of their "rights." A second reason is the residual fear that the National Board is trying to become a national licensing body.

To the first objection I say that the voluntary acceptance by the state boards of the results of examinations of superior quality will not endanger their states' rights. In fact, with the present universal concern over manpower shortages in medicine, recognition would help to preserve states' rights by counteracting the arguments of those who would centralize more authority in Washington. In answer to the second, I quote a statement made by Dr. John Hubbard in 1965, "Very frankly we want no part of the legal responsibility of licensing physicians, which is a duty and function we believe belongs to the states."

The fact that a state board will accept the license of another state whose standards are obviously inferior and refuses to accept a certificate based upon examinations of superior quality is indeed hard to understand. Meanwhile, despite its detractors, the National Board of Medical Examiners continues to insist upon quality and daily becomes a more influential force in medical education and testing.

Bibliography

American Medical Association. 1902. National Board of Medical Examiners. *J.A.M.A.* 38:108.
———. 1914. National Standard Requirement for Medical Practice. *J.A.M.A.* 63:951–52.
———. 1950. State Board Number. *J.A.M.A.* 143:450.
———. 1959. State Board Number. *J.A.M.A.* 155:457.
———. 1968. State Board Number. *J.A.M.A.* 204:1088.
Cowles, J. T. and Hubbard, J. P. 1952. A Comparative Study of Essay and Objective Examinations for Medical Students. *J. Med. Educ.* 27, Part 2.
———. 1954. Validity and Reliability of the New Objective Tests. *J. Med. Educ.* 29:30–34.
Crouch, T. H. and Hughes, F. J. 1965. A Pre-test Post-test Study of the Internship in Air Force and Army Hospitals. *A Conference Commemorating the 50th Anniversary of the National Board of Medical Examiners*, pp. 55–68. Philadelphia: National Board of Medical Examiners.
Dodson, J. A. 1906. National Examining Board. *J.A.M.A.* 47:877.

Hubbard, J. P. 1961. The Role of Examining Boards in Medical Education and in Qualification for Clinical Practice. *J. Med. Educ.* 36:94–102.

———. 1965. The Present Position of the National Board of Medical Examiners. *J.A.M.A.* 192:824–27.

———. 1968. Additional Methods of Testing Fitness to Practice. *Fed. Bull.* 55:151–59.

Hubbard, J. P. and Clemens, W. V. 1960. A Comparative Evaluation of Medical Schools. *J. Med. Educ.* 35:134–41.

Hubbard, J. P., Furlow, L. T. and Matson, D. D. 1967. An In-Training Examination for Residents as a Guide to Learning. *New Eng. J. Med.* 276:448–51.

Hubbard, J. P., Levit, E. J., Schumacher, C. F. and Schnabel, T. G. 1965. An Objective Evaluation of Clinical Competence. *New Eng. J. Med.* 272:1321–28.

Jason, H. 1965. Sequential Examinations in Assessing the Impact of a New Medical Curriculum. *A Conference Commemorating the 50th Anniversary of the National Board of Medical Examiners*, pp. 23–32. Philadelphia: National Board of Medical Examiners.

Levit, E. J. 1968. The Use of Motion Pictures in Evaluation of Fitness to Practice. *Fed. Bull.* 55:142–56.

Levit, E. J., Schumacher, C. F., and Hubbard, J. P. 1963. The Effect of Characteristics of Hospitals in Relation to the Caliber of Interns Obtained and the Competence of Interns After One Year of Training. *J. Med. Educ.* 38:909–19.

National Board of Medical Examiners. 1968. *National Board Examiner.* 15:7.

Rodman, W. L. 1915. Work of American Medical Association. *J.A.M.A.* 64:2107–15.

Womack, N. A. 1965. The Evolution of the National Board of Medical Examiners. *J.A.M.A.* 192:817–23.

CHAPTER SIX

LICENSING BOARDS AND DISCIPLINE

Without a doubt the most onerous duties demanded of members of boards of medical examiners lie in the field of medical discipline. The awesome responsibility of having to revoke the license of a physician, thus depriving him not only of a means of livelihood but also of his entire way of life, weighs heavily upon them. They also are acutely aware of their obligation to the public; regardless of their sympathy for the errant physician their primary responsibility is the safety of the patient.

Adding to the difficulties of boards in dealing with disciplinary problems is the fact that often they must assume the multiple roles of investigators, prosecutors, juries, judges, and executioners. In only a few states, such as California, are disciplinary matters investigated and presented to the boards by hearing officers. In all but two states—New York and Washington—the boards have disciplinary functions superimposed upon their examining and educational duties which, particularly in the larger states, can place an intolerable burden upon them. To add to the difficulties, the functions and powers of the boards are poorly understood both by the public and by the medical profession so that they are besieged by complaints which have no merit; nevertheless they may be castigated for lack of action. Many are the complainants who vanish when they learn that they might be called upon to testify at a hearing. Furthermore, few people have even rudimentary comprehension of due process under the law.

We must remember that the boards of medical examiners are legally constituted bodies of the state governments and as such they confine their activities to investigations of violations of the laws. Minor infractions of medical ethics or disputes between patients and doctors about fees do not concern the boards and are best referred to the local county societies or the hospital staffs.

To determine the magnitude of disciplinary problems and the types of offenses handled by the boards, I reviewed the actions taken by them for the five years from 1963 through 1967. My main source of information was the files of the Federation of State Medical Boards of the United States. Although the list may be incomplete, it does afford a broad view of the situation. Included in my tabulation are only definitive actions; I omitted cases in which prosecution was dropped for lack of evidence. Also excluded were the reports of cases in which former actions were rescinded and cancellation of licenses for technical reasons such as failure to pay registration fees.

From 1963 through 1967 I found that a total of 938 actions against physicians were taken by the boards. Table 4 reveals that the most common penalty was the imposition of probation, the second being the outright revocation of a license. However, before a licensee can be placed on probation, the license usually must first be revoked and then restored under certain terms and conditions. Furthermore, some of the revocations did not constitute original actions but resulted from violations of the terms of previous probations. The distribution throughout the years was fairly uniform.

Table 5 shows the reasons for action. It is obvious from this that some type of violation of the narcotics laws was by far the most common ground for discipline. The next most common was mental incompetence followed closely by fraud

Table 4. Types of Disciplinary Actions

Probation	375
Revocation	334
Suspension	161
Reprimands	68
Total	938

Table 5.   Causes for Disciplinary Actions

Narcotics	440
Mental Incompetence	94
Fraud and Deceit in Practice	74
Conviction of Felony	72
Abortions	71
Alcoholism	41
Unprofessional Conduct	68
Moral Turpitude	26
Gross Malpractice	7
Fraud in Application	6
Gross Immorality	3
Fee Splitting	1
Gross Misconduct	1

and deceit in the practice of medicine, the performance of criminal abortions, and unprofessional conduct; the last is often a general term covering many offenses. The 41 cases involving alcoholism may seem small in number but frequently this was associated with drug addiction. I have included under this category only those cases in which alcohol alone was mentioned. Some of the commonest causes for action deserve individual consideration.

As difficulties involving narcotics constituted such a large proportion of offenses—46 per cent—I classified these according to the types of violations. Table 6 gives this information. This of necessity is an arbitrary classification because these violators were often also guilty of unprofessional conduct or fraud. But because of the magnitude of the problem I concentrated upon the narcotics aspect which was mentioned as the primary cause of action. By far the largest number of violations were due to personal addiction of the physician. The second commonest problem, violation of the narcotics laws, varied in seriousness from mere technical offenses due to ignorance of the law or carelessness to flagrant violations of the laws such as failure to keep proper records of narcotics dispensed or prescribing of narcotics for known addicts. Eighteen of the actions were concerned with amphetamines and other dangerous

Table 6. Types of Narcotics Violations

Addiction	258
Violation of narcotics laws	65
Illegal prescribing	33
Prescribing for known addicts	23
Issuing false and fradulent prescriptions	21
Amphetamine, etc., peddling	18
Prescribing drugs without physical examination	11
Obtaining narcotics by fraud	9
Illegal sale	2
Total actions	440

drugs and usually involved their illegal sale by physicians; if these are subtracted from the total we find only 422 cases in which narcotics alone were involved.

While for a long time it has been common knowledge that the misuse of narcotics was one of the gravest hazards to physicians, only recently have the authorities directed much attention to the problem. One of the first to emphasize the danger in recent years was Glaspel (1958) who devoted his entire presidential address before the Federation of State Medical Boards to narcotics addiction among physicians. He pointed out that of 3,000 addicts admitted to the United States Public Health Service Hospital in Lexington, Kentucky, each year, 50 are physicians. Among the general population in the United States there is one addict to 3,000 people; among the physician population the proportion is one to 100. Said Glaspel, "To state it another more dramatic way, enough doctors to equal the entire annual output of one of our medical schools degenerates into addiction each year." What a waste!

Jones (1958), also of the Federation, described the problem of addiction among physicians in California. There, as in other states, the members of the Board of Medical Examiners firmly believe that one of their most important functions is to salvage and rehabilitate the addict if this can be done without endangering the public. California has led the other states in the handling of addicts and has established an elaborate system of probation which is regarded as a model by other state boards. But, before deciding upon the penalty for an offender, the board considers the following: the approximate length of time the physician has used narcotics; the amount of the drug taken; the duration of abstinence prior to the hearing before the board; and whether he has received any treatment for his addiction. If the board believes that there is a good chance that the physician addict can be rehabilitated it spells out the terms of probation in careful detail. The first step is surrender of the narcotics stamp. The physician must then place himself in the hands of a psychiatrist approved by the board. The board demands frequent reports of progress from the psychiatrist and in addition the probationer is required to report to the board at frequent intervals for interviews. Because of the fact that at all times there are over 100 physicians under surveillance, the probationers are divided among the board members so that they may receive individual attention and counsel.

Jones in 1958 reported that during the preceding ten years the California Board considered 138 cases involving addiction to narcotics in physicians. Eight licenses were revoked outright, eight were subsequently revoked for violation of the terms of probation, while three physicians were again called before the board and given additional terms of probation for minor infractions. Of 130 physicians placed on probation between 1948 and 1957, 41 successfully completed probation and were restored to good standing and 62 were still on probation. Jones claimed that the rehabilitation rate was 92 per cent. These results are at sharp variance with those of Wall (1958), who studied the outcome of hospital treatment in 44 physician addicts who were patients from 1927 to 1957. Of these, only 12 had been off the drug for from one to 29 years. Of the remaining 32, four committed suicide; the remainder were under treatment intermittently and were unable to work. Wall pointed out that the medical schools might help to prevent narcotics problems among physicians by including in their curricula proper instruction in the dangers that physicians face from drug addiction.

Putnam and Ellinwood (1966) also take a pessimistic view concerning the future of physicians addicted to narcotics. They pointed out that there were few satisfactory studies of physicians after they had been released from hospitals. Their study compared 68 male physician addicts discharged from the United States Public Health Service Hospital in Lexington, Kentucky with a control group of physicians matched for ages and geographic distribution in the American Medical Association Directory of Physicians. They found that the attrition rate (those dropping out of practice) was 21 per cent for the control group and 43 per cent among the addicts. They also found that the patients moved from one location to another twice as frequently as did the controls.

Obviously there is wide variation in the rates of relapse among different groups of physician addicts. Satisfactory rehabilitation varies from a rate of 27 per cent to the 92 per cent reported by the California board. A possible explanation is that the group with the lowest incidence of rehabilitation was composed of hardened addicts when they began treatment. On the other hand, the California series is made up of selected physicians whose addiction was of short duration and who entered treatment early. Another consideration is the fact that Wall followed his patients longer. Nevertheless the results in California do appear encouraging.

Drug addiction in physicians has been called an occupational disease. One finds various explanations for this all based upon the ready availability of drugs. The main reasons given for addiction are fatigue, physical illness, and strain of practicing medicine caused by the great responsibility of the doctor. None of these explanations is satisfactory. The typical physician addict, when called before a board of medical examiners and asked how he happened to become addicted, will offer an explanation such as the following: "I had a large practice which forced me to work long hours; this brought about a constant state of fatigue. One night when I was unusually tired and could not sleep I gave myself an injection of demerol (or morphine). This made me feel so much better that I soon tried it again and the next thing I knew I was 'hooked'."

Some addicts will say that they had painful physical illnesses so that they were forced to give themselves narcotics. The only trouble with this is that by the time the physician addict is called before the board the illness might no longer exist but the addiction remains. Psychiatrists tell us that very few serious addictions result from administration of narcotics for pain only.

Furthermore, to obtain the drugs to satisfy the addiction the physician must resort with ever increasing frequency to fraudulent practices. Therefore, the fact that a physician would knowingly administer a dangerous and addicting drug to himself calls for a much more logical explanation than that he is tired or in pain. He should be aware of the well known fact that he must never take narcotics except under the direction of a fellow physician. One can only conclude that the doctor who administers narcotics to himself does so either without regard for the consequences or because of ignorance. As neither of these explanations is logical, one can only conclude that his addiction is a manifestation of a deep personality disorder or of mental illness.

Wall (1958) attempted to delineate the personality type of the addict. He found that in his series half of them had mentally ill relatives in the preceding generation. He stated that, unlike the alcoholic, the addict had no close attachments to parents or siblings during childhood. Said Wall, "The outstanding personality traits were sensitive tendermindedness with a tendency toward hypochondriasis, to tire easily, and inability to stand life when the going was hard." Significant is the fact that in Wall's series of 44 physician addicts, 28 exhibited immaturity, irresponsibility, and unreliability, traits found in the psychopathic personality; 12 had past histories of depression, while four were schizoid.

Jones (1967) unequivocally defined the psychopathology of the physician addict. He said that narcotic addiction was a "clinically valid psychiatric entity, namely a depression." He continued, "Aside from depressive symptomatology and good results from depressive treatment regimens, such as electroshock therapy, a good case for a depressive etiology of narcotic addiction of physicians can be made by longitudinal studies of common personality traits and psychodynamic factors." His thesis is further bolstered by the fact that among 31 cases which he studied there were six suicides.

Grave as is the problem of narcotics addiction among physicians, there is at least one encouraging note; most of the state boards are facing it firmly and they are trying to rehabilitate the addicts whenever possible. As they acquire further knowledge their efforts should become more successful. In addition it is possible that more reliable methods of psychological evaluation will be developed which will enable the admissions committees of the medical schools to evaluate their candidates more effectively and to eliminate those with depressive personality traits.

The second most common disciplinary problem, incompetence due to mental illness, is indeed complicated. Its causes are as varied as its manifestations. They range from organic brain disease causing rapid deterioration of judgement and memory, which are obvious to the most casual observer, to lesser personality disorders which, though they might cause temporary impairment of judgement, are reversible. The situation is further complicated by the fact that there are varying degrees of normality and, no matter how dangerous a mentally ill physician may be, he is often not committable and his errors can be considered due to mere eccentricity rather than to illness. Over a hundred years ago Herman Melville aptly pointed out this delicate balance when he said, "Who in the rainbow can draw the line where the violet tint ends and the orange begins? Distinctly we see the difference of the colors, but where exactly does the one first blendingly enter into the other? So with sanity and insanity. . . ."

For a long time few laws mentioned incompetence due to mental illness as a cause for disciplinary action. Obviously a physician, while he is incarcerated in a mental hospital, is not dangerous to the public; but in many states the laws place no limitations upon the practice of the physician after he has been released from the hospital. Furthermore, they make no provision for the important aspects of rehabilitation. In 1960 I conducted a survey of the attitudes of the state boards toward mental illness among physicians. I found that the problem was specifically mentioned in the laws of only 27 states. In 17 states commitment to an institution constituted grounds for automatic revocation or suspension of a license, while in nine the license could be revoked only after a hearing. In only 11 states was there any policy established either by law or regulation to assist the mentally ill in rehabilitation. But the boards were probably not as heartless as one might conclude because an additional 16 states provided for probation which might help in rehabilitation (Derbyshire, 1960).

In 1966 Merchant determined the number of state laws which had been amended since 1960 to include mental illness in physicians. He discovered that 12 more states had included mental illness specifically in their laws which brought the total number to 39. In addition, he found that six more state boards had made rules and regulations concerning the handling of mentally ill physicians and that eight more had established a policy of assisting them. Merchant concluded, "There remains an appreciable area in which such recognition of the problem is unresolved and conclusions drawn from the 1960 report still obtain today—nevertheless it is encouraging to see further progress in the past five years."

California again leads the way in its methods of dealing with mental illness. Its law is designed both to protect the public and to aid the mentally ill physician. In part the California law (1967) reads, "Before reinstating such a person (one who has been mentally ill) the board may require the person to pass an oral or written examination or both, to determine fitness to resume practice." Furthermore, the board may require him to obtain additional training, to submit to a complete diagnostic examination by one or more physicians appointed by the board, and to restrict the scope or type of practice. See State of California Business and Professions Code Sec. 2415–2419, 2618, 2689, 2964.

Mentally ill physicians who have not reached the stage of legal commitment to an institution constitute a danger all of their own. No law has yet been devised to deal with them satis-

84

factorily without infringing upon their constitutional rights. The legislatures will probably never grant the boards arbitrary power to prosecute such individuals and they should not. Therefore, until a fair and reasonable legal approach can be devised, they are best controlled by the hospitals in which they practice.

The third commonest ground for disciplinary action listed in Table 5, fraud and deceit in the practice of medicine, often resulted only in formal reprimands. Many of these cases occurred in a period of two years in one of the larger states in which there was a conspiracy among a ring of unscrupulous lawyers and doctors to defraud insurance companies. At first glance the penalty appears mild but I do not know all of the circumstances.

The fourth most common offense, conviction of a felony, requires little discussion as the boards acted only after decisions had been made by the courts. In most cases the boards could exercise no discretion and were forced to revoke the licenses of the defendants automatically. I found an exception in the case of income tax evasion. Here there was no uniformity, the penalities ranging from revocation to reprimand. In 1960 Deal reported the results of a questionnaire sent to state boards from which he learned that 13 states were not concerned about this offense. His own conclusion: "Being mindful that the existing legal punishment for income tax evasion . . . is very harsh . . . I am not convinced that the severe punitive program should be augmented in every case . . . by forfeiture of a physician's right to practice."

The commission of criminal abortion, while also a felony, is placed in a separate category because it was given as grounds for action in 71 cases. This is one offense concerning which the boards seem to be in complete agreement (Gundry, 1960). The penalty is almost always revocation although suspension was mentioned by three state boards.

Unprofessional conduct was given as the cause for action in 68 cases. The penalties varied from reprimand to revocation of licenses. Unprofessional conduct is defined in many state laws but in some instances such a charge may act as a catch-all when a board is convinced that disciplinary action should be taken but that the crime does not fit neatly into another category. The definition of unprofessional conduct, as given in Black's Law Dictionary, is, "that which is by general opinion considered to be grossly unprofessional because immoral or dishonorable—that which violates the ethical code of the profession as such conduct which is unbecoming in a member of a profession in good standing."

Holman (1961) made a study of the laws of all of the states as they applied to unprofessional conduct. He found more than 90 grounds for revocation or suspension of a license. Moreover he learned that no one ground, stated in the same words, was to be found in all of the statutes and that the laws of no state contained all grounds. Nine grounds were found repeated in 30 or more laws. These were: drug addiction, unprofessional conduct, fraud in connection with examination or licensure, alcoholism, advertising, performance of criminal abortions, conviction of felonies, conviction of offenses involving moral turpitude, and mental incapacity. Although an offense might appear to constitute unprofessional conduct, defense attorneys have often successfully argued that the defendant physician should be absolved because his specific offense is not enumerated in the law.

Holman concluded, "Because of the present lack of uniformity, each state must 'go it alone,' building up its own body of law slowly and painstakingly. Frequently it is necessary to determine judicially whether the act complained of is actually an offense within the meaning and under the language of the particular statute involved."

Terry, formerly judge of the Superior Court of Delaware, pointed to the dilemma of many boards when he referred to the doctor who does something dubious without being called to task for it because of the fact that the legality or the propriety of his act is doubtful. He emphasized that standards should be spelled out. He said that without well-defined standards enforcement is retarded. Equally important, enforcement without adequate standards produces injustice (Terry, 1962).

One of the most vexing problems facing the state boards is not commonly found in the lists of grounds for discipline; this is professional incompetence. In 1965 I studied this situation. I found several forms of incompetence recognized. Ranked in order of frequency, they are mental, professional, physical, and the form due to ignorance or stupidity. My study was based upon questionnaires that I directed to the state medical societies and upon perusal of all of the medical practice laws. The constitutions and bylaws of 38 state medical societies did not specify incompetence as a cause for action against their members. In the states which did have such provisions, members could be expelled for incompetence. But only seven societies had ever disciplined physicians because of incompetence.

The laws of only 27 states specifically mentioned mental incompetence as a reason for action, while 18 laws provided for action because of physical or professional incompetence. (The latter was defined as the inability to practice medicine by modern methods.) The only semblance of uniformity was found in the laws of seven states which in general provided that a license could be revoked if there is "any physical or mental disability which renders the further practice of medicine by the licensee dangerous." In other states the incompetent physician apparently cannot be deterred by law until after he has caused grievous injury to a patient; at least so one would infer from reading their laws which state that gross malpractice resulting in the death of a patient is a reason for revocation (Derbyshire, 1965).

The American Medical Association has become vitally interested in the problems involving incompetence. This was emphasized by Dr. James Appel, a past president, who stated that on the whole the boards of medical examiners had satisfactorily performed their duty of deciding who should be initially allowed to practice medicine. But he pointed out that organized medicine has not been zealous enough in checking on continuing competence. He said, "One of our major objectives now is to stimulate greater emphasis on insuring

competence and observance of law and ethics *after* licensure''
(Appel, 1966).

In 1966 Regan reported on the handling of the physically
incompetent physician. In regard to congenital defects he
suggested that they should be noted and assessed when a
student applies for admission to medical school. If he is accepted in spite of such defects he should be guided into a field
in which they would handicap him least and not endanger his
patients. He applied the same suggestion to acquired defects.

I am astonished at the large number of hospitals which do
not require a certificate of competence from the physician who
has presumably recovered from a serious physical illness before
he resumes his practice. His affliction may vary from coronary
thrombosis to a minor stroke. In any case he may be welcomed
back to duty without demand of adequate proof of his ability
to function normally. Regan suggested that as an additional
safeguard the hospital bylaws provide that staff members be
required to submit reports of physical examinations at specific
ages. This is another example of a problem which the hospitals
can handle much better than can the boards of medical examiners. But I am not implying that medical practice acts should
not contain provisions for action in cases of proven professional,
physical, or mental incompetence. Although in such cases the
hospital staffs should be primarily concerned, they should know
that they will be supported by law if necessary. Particularly
important is the law in prosecuting the renegade physician who
belongs to neither hospital staff nor medical society but who
victimizes his patients in his office.

A recent decision of the Kansas Supreme Court, discussed
in detail in another chapter, may help to clarify the issue of
incompetence when it is not specifically mentioned in the law.
A district court had reversed the order of the board of medical
examiners because the statute did not list incompetency as a
specific act constituting unprofessional conduct. In overruling
the decision of the lower court, the Supreme Court stated that
the object of the statute was to protect the public from incompetent practitioners and that therefore the board was not
wrong in taking such action.

From the foregoing discussion it is obvious that disciplinary problems in medicine run the gamut in complexity from imprisonment of a felon to violation of the fine points of medical ethics over which the board might not have jurisdiction. The boards, as agents of the state governments, are primarily concerned with violations of the law, although other lesser offenses can still cause danger to the public. In regard to the latter, approved hospitals are assuming an ever increasing position of importance. The least active bodies in discipline are the local medical societies whose powers are limited. But they can provide much help in the prosecution of malefactors.

In 1960 the American Medical Association became concerned about the enforcement of medical discipline. It appointed a committee which investigated the problem exhaustively by means of a series of meetings throughout the entire United States. Dr. Raymond M. McKeowen, its chairman, summarized the conclusions as follows: 1. The committee believed that in the matter of discipline the principle of states' rights is paramount—each state has the responsibility to care for its own problems through available channels. 2. Most boards of medical examiners are inadequately financed to do the job they would like to do. 3. Although most state medical societies reported that disciplinary mechanisms were adequate, this was not always the case. 4. Little was being done by either medical societies or boards of medical examiners to report their activities in the field of discipline (McKeowen, 1961). As a result of the work of the committee, today there is better reporting of disciplinary actions; the constitution and bylaws of the American Medical Association were amended to provide for "original jurisdiction" by the Judicial Council in cases in which the local societies refused to act. To date this power has been used sparingly.

Various estimates have been made of the proportion of unscrupulous, unethical, delinquent, and incompetent physicians among the population; these have varied from two to ten per cent. Perhaps five per cent is a fair figure, although it can be only a rough estimate. But even this small number poses a grave danger because of the responsibilities of physicians for human welfare and lives. Therefore, it is imperative that all agencies concerned—the hospitals, the medical societies, and the boards of medical examiners—stand united in their efforts to enforce discipline in the medical profession and to protect the public against the depredations of the malefactors.

Bibliography

Appel, J. Z. 1966. Eleventh Annual Walter L. Bierring Lecture. *Fed. Bull.* 53:66–74.

Black's Law Dictionary. 4th ed. 1957. St. Paul, Minnesota: West Publishing Co.

Deal, A. M. 1960. Study of Attitudes and Opinions of State Boards of Medical Examiners Regarding Income Tax Evasion and Other Felonies. *Fed. Bull.* 47:404–408.

Derbyshire, R. C. 1960. Current Attitudes Towards Mental Illness in Physicians. *Fed. Bull.* 47:352–58.

———. 1965. What Should the Profession Do About the Incompetent Physician? *J.A.M.A.* 194:119–22.

Glaspel, C. J. 1958. Problems in Narcotic Addiction. *Fed. Bull.* 45:200–207.

Gundry, L. P. 1960. Current Attitudes in Discipline: Abortions. *Fed. Bull.* 47:378–80.

Holman, E. J. 1961. The Complex of Unprofessional Conduct. *Fed. Bull.* 48:58–69.

Jones, C. H. 1967. Narcotic Addiction of Physicians. *Northwest Med.* 66:555–64.

Jones, L. E. 1958. Experience With Probation in California. *Fed. Bull.* 45:165–73.

McKeowen, R. M. 1961. Present Status of Medical Discipline. *Fed. Bull.* 38:132–41.

Merchant, F. T. 1966. Mental Illness: A Follow-up. *Fed. Bull.* 53:282–97.

Putnam, P. L. and Ellinwood, E. H., Jr. 1966. Narcotics Addiction Among Physicians: A Ten Year Follow-up. *Amer. J. Psychiat.* 122:745–48.

Regan, J. F. 1966. Physical Disability and Professional Incompetence. *Fed. Bull.* 53:318–30.

Terry, C. L. 1962. The Physician as a Defendant in Discipline. *Fed. Bull.* 49:85–95.

Wall, J. H. 1958. The Results of Hospital Treatment of Addiction in Physicians. *Fed. Bull.* 45:144–52.

CHAPTER SEVEN

STATE BOARDS AND THE COURTS

Misunderstandings concerning the legal aspects of medical practice may give rise to accusations that boards of medical examiners are derelict in their duties. Disgruntled patients, believing that they have been wronged by their physicians, demand that boards revoke their licenses. Many of these complaints are not even within the jurisdiction of the boards, which are primarily concerned with violations of the law. Moreover, ignorance of the medical practice laws and of the responsibilities of the boards is not limited to the public; many doctors seem to believe that a medical license can be revoked merely because they personally dislike the individual who holds it. Physicians may make loose accusations undocumented by evidence; often when asked to reduce their charges to writing, or if they are requested to appear as witnesses in a hearing, they hastily withdraw their charges, though they may continue to mutter about the unwillingness of the board to prosecute offenders. To guarantee that a physician will not be deprived of his license illegally, board decisions are subject to review by the courts. Although this helps to guarantee that a physician will not be deprived of his license illegally, the system carries with it the danger that a physician whose license ought to be revoked might be permitted to continue practicing for many months during which his case is being reviewed.

Let us assume that a state board of medical examiners, after a long and exhaustive hearing, has revoked the license of a physician. After carefully weighing the evidence, the board members have reluctantly reached the conclusion that the defendant physician is guilty as charged and that if he is not removed from the practice of medicine he will continue to be a danger both to the public and to himself. The board members, men of good will, torn between their reluctance to banish a colleague and the realization that their primary duty is to the public, are emotionally exhausted. Despite the unpleasantness of their jobs they believe that they have done their work well. But what happens? Within the next two or three days they receive an order from the court staying their verdict pending formal appeal. The guilty doctor is allowed to continue to practice despite the fact that his license has been revoked.

No matter how searching the deliberations of any board, its action can be reversed by the court. The defendant physician has the right to appeal any decision. In an action as serious as revocation of a license the decision of the board cannot be the last word. Boards cannot be allowed to take arbitrary and capricious actions, but some reversals may be based upon technicalities, thus allowing a dangerous person to continue to prey upon the public. All too frequently, as in our hypothetical case, the court will grant a stay order against the board so that in essence it substitutes its judgement for that of experienced members of the board who might be much more fit to judge the technical aspects of the case than is the court. In these days of crowded dockets this might entail a delay of months before the court is able to hear the case. If the case finally goes to the state supreme court the delay can easily stretch out into two or three years. Aside from the damage that the guilty physician can do pending a final decision by the court, the board can be placed in an unfavorable position in the eyes of the public. In fact, the question is often raised as to whether or not the medical profession is adequately policing its ranks as it claims to do.

The functions of the courts in regard to disciplinary actions of state boards vary widely throughout the United States. In some states the appeal is heard *de novo*—that is, the case is tried all over again by the court. In others the case may be heard by a jury; in still other states the court merely reviews the record of the hearing to be sure that the accused has not been deprived of his rights and to determine whether or not proper procedures have been followed and whether the board has acted arbitrarily or capriciously. The courts are particularly interested in making sure that the defendant has not been deprived of "due process" under the Fourteenth Amendment to the Constitution of the United States. The 1967 *Disciplinary Digest* of the American Medical Association points out that the police power of the states has certain limitations. "The due process clause of the Fourteenth Amendment to the U.S. Constitution, other constitutional provisions, and state constitutional provisions, perpetuate the social values which are the fibre of our democratic system by shielding the basic rights of citizens from official abuse. The Fourteenth Amendment reads in part: 'No state shall . . . deprive any person of life, liberty or property without due process of law.' " The license to practice medicine is considered a privilege by some, while others maintain it is a property right; nevertheless, revocation of a license deprives a physician of his means of livelihood and is not to be undertaken lightly. Therefore, the courts hold that a license can be revoked only in a constitutionally acceptable manner. The *Disciplinary Digest* (1967) states, "Thus, courts hold that statutes providing for the revocation or suspension of licenses must specify the conduct for which sanctions can be imposed."

How frequently are decisions of the boards of medical examiners overruled by the courts? In 1963, C. Joseph Stetler, then chief legal counsel of the American Medical Association, addressed the Federation of State Medical Boards on this subject. He found that during the five-year period from 1957 through 1961 there were only three reversals. He complimented the boards when he said, "It is interesting for attorneys to note the ability of the boards of medical examiners to sift through superficialities and to arrive at proper legislative conclusions despite their lack of training in the law." However, since Stetler's study, either the boards have lost their legal acumen or the defendant physicians have become more litigious. I found that in the five-year period from 1963 through 1967 the courts overruled board actions 15 times.

The Law Division of the American Medical Association, in 1967, published its valuable "Disciplinary Digest." It contains a large collection of court decisions regarding disciplinary actions of state boards. Included are decisions which have been upheld as well as those which have been reversed. The cases cover a long period of time, extending from 1902 through 1966; 251 cases are included. In 74 of these or 29 per cent the courts have ruled against the boards. Another publication of the American Medical Association, "The Citation," also analyzes court decisions concerning boards. Here (A.M.A., 1967) I found four additional cases in which the courts have overruled board actions since 1966, bringing the total of adverse decisions to 78. Although my list is probably not complete, it affords an idea of the frequency of reversals as well as the reasons. In the *Digest* the types of cases are broken down into three broad categories, "Constitutional Considerations," "The Offense," and "Procedural Matters."

Under the heading, "Constitutional Considerations," we learn the troubles which boards have with the offense, unprofessional conduct, discussed in detail in another chapter. For example, a statute of the District of Columbia provides for disciplinary action in case a physician is found guilty of "unprofessional or dishonorable conduct." The court held that this was too vague and uncertain to be capable of enforcement because it did not provide advance notice to physicians practicing their profession of the acts for which their right to practice might be taken away. Said the court, "The underlying question involved in all cases that may arise is whether the courts can uphold and enforce a statute whose broad and indefinite language may apply not only to a particular act about which there might be radical differences, thereby devolving upon the tribunals charged with enforcement of the law the exercise of an arbitrary power of discriminating between the several classes of acts" (the Czarra case, 1925).

On the other hand, in a Washington case the court ruled that charges of unprofessional conduct against a physician were not void for uncertainty since the several subdivisions of the statute defined specific conduct to which the term "unprofessional conduct" could be applied (State Board of Medical Examiners v. Macy [1916]).

Members of boards of medical examiners are often embarrassed by the insistence of the courts that proper procedures be carried out. They may be baffled when the courts overrule them on the basis of what they consider unimportant technicalities. But procedure is important and failure to follow it may deprive the accused of due process. This is illustrated by an Arizona case where a physician received a notice stating that his license to practice medicine would be suspended if he did not appear and answer charges on a specified date. As a result of evidence produced at the hearing the doctor's license was revoked. The court held that the physician's right to notice embraced not only the accusations against him but the contemplated disciplinary action as well. The court ruled that the board could not change its mind and decide to revoke rather than to suspend once the proceedings were under way (Board of Medical Examiners v. Schutzbank, 1963).

Today almost all medical practice laws list in detail the acts which are considered to constitute unprofessional conduct. However, it is impossible to foresee and define every such act and on many occasions decisions of boards have been overruled because the particular dereliction was not enumerated in the statute. A notable exception to this was a recent ruling of the Supreme Court of Kansas. The Board of the Healing Arts revoked a physician's license for "extreme incompetency" in the treatment of patients under his care. The charges were supported by expert witnesses as well as by hospital records which showed a consistent pattern of incompetence and utter disregard of the welfare of his patients. The Board ruled that his incompetency constituted unprofessional conduct.

A trial court reversed the Board's order because the statute authorizing revocation of a physician's license for unprofessional conduct did not list incompetency as a cause for action. The Board appealed to the Supreme Court which reinstated the revocation order and ruled that the Board had not exceeded its authority and had not unlawfully created a new ground for revocation as alleged by the trial court. The Supreme Court said, "It would indeed be difficult not to say impractical, in carrying out the purpose of the act, for the legislature to list each and every specific act or course of conduct which might constitute such unprofessional conduct of a disqualifying nature. Nor does any such failure leave the statute subject to attack on grounds of vagueness or indefiniteness—no conduct or practice could be more devastating to the health and welfare of a patient or the public than incompetency; integral to the whole policy the legislature had in mind must be the power of the board to protect against it." A fundamental feature of the decision of the Supreme Court was incorporated in comments regarding the original appeal to the lower court. It ruled that the trial court weighed the evidence and made "de novo findings of fact and substituted its judgement for that of the board, which it was not authorized to do" (American Medical Association, *The Citation*, 1967).

Occasionally bewildering to boards are some court decisions concerning specific offenses. One of these is advertising which is frowned upon in all respectable medical circles. But the courts might have other opinions, as in the Colorado case in which a physician visited various parts of the state advertising his activities and pointing to his ability to treat certain diseases. The Board of Medical Examiners revoked his license for unprofessional conduct. But, strangely enough, the court annulled the revocation on the grounds that advertising is not unprofessional conduct unless it is dishonorable in the common judgement of mankind. The court observed that medical ethics are standards of behavior imposed by physicians. It held that charges of unprofessional conduct were not proved by evidence that the doctor had advertised in such a manner as was prohibited by the principles of medical ethics (Sapero v. State Board of Medical Examiners, 1932).

Board members also may be baffled by some court decisions regarding fraud. I found several such cases; one striking one occurred in New York (the Rosen case, 1962). The Board of Regents, the disciplinary body of that state, found minor discrepancies between medical reports submitted in personal injury cases and testimony of patients called as witnesses. The doctor had destroyed all of the history cards of patients referred by one lawyer, and proof that the physician had given an attorney blank bills or statements to be typed was held to be no more than suspicious circumstances and did not justify a finding of fraud and deceit in the practice of medicine. Another court decision which must have puzzled the board occurred in Colorado. The board found that a physician was guilty of conduct detrimental to the public in claiming medical qualifications, degrees, and special training which he did not have or which were of no recognized value. The court, in overruling the revocation order of the board, observed that the state does not require any additional license or certification for a physician who practices a specialty and that licensure by the board entitles a licensee to practice medicine in all of its branches (Colorado State Board of Medical Examiners v. Weiler, 1965).

For many years there were few definite rules governing board hearings and any procedure which was considered orderly was acceptable. But this is not the case today; almost all the states have passed laws which prescribe elaborate procedures that must be followed to the letter from the original notice of contemplated action through all phases of the hearing, findings of fact, and the decision of the board. As all boards must be thoroughly acquainted with the rules of procedure, their actions should not be reversed because of failure to abide by them. Therefore, it was surprising to find 33 such instances. Some of the errors obviously could have been avoided. For example, in one case a board failed to provide specific findings of fact in the record. The physician was charged with four specific acts of misconduct. But the court found that, in view of the omissions, it was impossible to determine whether the board found the physician guilty as to all of the charges. Although the action of the board was not reversed, the case was remanded to have the board enter the necessary findings of fact (State Board of Medical Examiners v. Gandy, 1966). In another case the error occurred during the hearing when the board refused a physician the right to examine copies of investigator's reports and to cross examine the investigator as to their contents. The revocation was annulled because cross-examination was unduly restricted (Rothenberg v. Board of Regents of the University of the State of New York, 1943).

Despite the fact that both the boards and the courts must make every effort to be fair to physicians accused of professional misconduct, one views with alarm the long delays involved in appeals of board decisions. When a physician's license has been revoked the court may issue a stay order against the board pending a court decision; therefore, a dangerous person can continue to prey upon the public for many months.

A long delay caused by the difficulty in obtaining sufficient evidence against wrongdoers and compounded by the slow pace of the courts is exemplified by a recent New Mexico case. The questionable conduct of two physicians had been under scrutiny by the board of medical examiners and by the medical society for several years, but no clear-cut evidence of law violations could be obtained. Finally, however, a pattern of conduct of the physicians emerged which permitted the board to bring against them well-documented charges of fraud. After a hearing, the board revoked their licenses. The defendant physicians appealed to the district court, which promptly granted a stay of the board's order. This was later followed by the court's reversing the board's action. The board then appealed to the state Supreme Court, which, in turn, reversed the decision of the lower court and upheld the action of the board. Meanwhile the accused doctors, by court order, were permitted to practice medicine for some 23 months after the revocation of their licences.

An extreme example of the dangers which can result from such delays is the case of Dr. Ronald E. Clark of Michigan. I tell his story in some detail to illustrate not only the legal snarls in which the boards of medical examiners can become involved but also the disasters which can follow if a board is too lenient because its members allow a malefactor to play upon their sympathies.

The story of Dr. Clark, spanning a period of 11 years, begins on February 28, 1956. On that date the Michigan Board of Registration in Medicine revoked his license on the basis of moral turpitude and abortion, according to the report of the board. Later an article in the *Detroit News* (June 19, 1968) stated that the action was also taken because he molested women patients. Although this should have promptly ended the medical career of Dr. Clark, unfortunately there is much more to the story.

On June 6, 1956 Dr. Clark was arrested for practicing medicine without a license. Although the arrest was apparently based upon firm evidence, I was unable to determine the disposition of the charges. Nevertheless, on March 7, 1957, for reasons known only to its members, the Michigan Board restored his license on condition that he continue psychiatric treatment and report to the board every six months.

Dr. Clark next met with the Board on June 12, 1958 when his license was revoked for noncompliance with the terms of his probation. He appealed this action to the Ingham County Circuit Court which reversed the order of revocation and remanded the case to the board for another hearing. On December 5, 1958, at still another hearing, the Michigan Board revoked his license on the basis of commitment to a state mental hospital and on charges of assault upon a patient. On September 9, 1959, presumably after Dr. Clark had been released from the state hospital, the Ingham County Court again reversed the order of revocation and remanded the case back to the Board for still another hearing. On October 5, 1959, the Board again revoked his license for unprofessional and dishonest conduct and moral turpitude. Apparently the defendant's old weakness had reappeared, as the specific offense was "taking indecent liberties with person of woman in his office." But the revocation order was stayed pending appeal to the Ingham County Circuit Court. Therefore, Dr. Clark was able to continue his practice for over a year until August 11, 1961 when the Circuit Court affirmed the order of the Board. Did this stop him from practicing his profession? By no means.

On August 31, 1961 the Board was served with an injunction staying its decision pending Dr. Clark's appeal to the Supreme Court of Michigan. About a year later, in a lengthy decision which incidentally reviewed the previous actions, the Supreme Court affirmed the 1961 order of the Circuit Court upholding the October 1959 order of the Board.

99

But even the Supreme Court decision did not end the story of Dr. Clark. The Board of Registration granted his request for one more hearing and on October 3, 1963 it restored his license to practice medicine. No doubt the Board considered that he no longer had psychopathic propensities because his conduct while awaiting the last decision indicated that he had become a useful member of society. But obviously this conclusion was wrong. Dr. Clark next came to the attention of the public when headlines in the *New York Times* of December 3, 1967 announced, "9 Deaths Studied in Doctor's Case." According to the article, Dr. Ronald Clark had been charged in the death of Mrs. Grace Neil, his part time office assistant who died in his office on November 3, 1967. At autopsy it was found that she died from an overdose of pentothal sodium which he had used to treat her heart disease—unorthodox treatment to say the least. The arrest of Dr. Clark followed a dramatic 12-hour chase through the snow in five-degree weather by the police who were led by a bloodhound.

Meanwhile the prosecutor was investigating a "large incidence of deaths attributed to therapeutic misadventure, cardiac arrest, or an injection of one sort or another."

At last, in July, 1968 Dr. Clark was effectively removed from the practice of medicine when he was convicted of manslaughter and sentenced to three to 15 years in prison. Let us hope that his license has been permanently revoked by now. But the public furor has not subsided by any means. A recent article in *Medical World News* stated that medical licensing in Michigan will become a political football partly due to a blast at the Board of Registration by the prosecuting attorney of Oakland County. In a public statement he claimed that the death of Dr. Clark's nurse would never have occurred had not the medical profession been anxious to protect its own. He called upon the legislature to strengthen the licensing procedures and suggested the addition of a layman to the Board.

How can one explain the fantastic tale of Dr. Clark? How could a board of medical examiners bring itself to restore a license which had been revoked for abortion, moral turpitude, and molesting female patients? And this after he had been previously arrested for practicing medicine without a license? Was it due to extreme compassion of the board members for an erring fellow physician? No doubt during the 11-year period covering Dr. Clark's relations with the Board there were several changes of personnel. Is it possible that the new members of the board were inclined to be too lenient?

An appalling feature of the case is that due to the numerous delays by the courts this obviously dangerous man was permitted to practice for a total of almost three years after his license had been revoked. It is no easier to account for the slow pace of the courts than for the compassion of the Board in restoring his license on two occasions. This is a prime example of the danger of the court substituting its judgement for that of the board, which it did by staying the orders of the board and permitting the man to continue to practice. No doubt the Board members reasoned that it was permissible to restore his license as the courts obviously did not consider it dangerous for him to continue to practice.

According to the *New York Times* there was another reason for the compassion of the Board; Dr. Clark pled poverty. However, another news source said that his license was restored because he swore that he was going to Ghana permanently as a medical missionary. Whether or not his plan to toil in the vineyard of the Lord was serious I cannot say; but obviously he was soon back in Michigan to resume his depredations upon an unsuspecting public.

Some serious lessons evolve from the story of Dr. Clark. First, if the crime of a physician is so heinous as to justify the outright revocation of his license, it should never be restored. The Michigan Board must have rued the day that it reopened Dr. Clark's case for reconsideration. In the case of lesser derelictions, suspension or probation can be used. Secondly, something should be done to prevent the courts from substituting their judgement for that of the Board by granting stay orders when licenses have been revoked. If, in the interest of justice, a stay order must be issued, then let the court hear the case promptly no matter how crowded its docket. Thirdly, boards of medical examiners should realize that a medical license cannot with safety be restored on condition that a physician go far away, even to Ghana. No license can be restored under such a condition. So there was nothing to prevent Dr. Clark from legally resuming his practice in Michigan. Finally there must be a limit to the compassion of board members. In hindsight they should have been more concerned with the safety of the public than with the plea of poverty of Dr. Clark. After all, he could have found another way of earning a living; he might even have driven a taxi. The whole affair is preposterous.

That the Supreme Court of at least one state was concerned about a court substituting its judgement for that of the board was illustrated by a recent decision in New Mexico. The Board of Medical Examiners revoked the licenses of two physicians for dishonorable and unprofessional conduct when it found them guilty of fraud in the practice of medicine. The physicians promptly appealed to the District Court which issued a stay order against the Board pending a formal hearing. After disqualification of three judges, the appeal was finally heard by the Court. The Court reversed the decision of the Board on the basis that there was not clear and convincing evidence to support the allegations, the decision of the Board was unsupported by substantial evidence, and the Board acted arbitrarily and capriciously.

The New Mexico Board of Medical Examiners appealed to the Supreme Court. Some 21 months after the initial revocation of the physicians' licenses, the decision of the lower court was reversed. Significant was the final comment of the Supreme Court: "The record in the instant case supports the Board's decision by clear and convincing evidence and the decision of the Board is neither unreasonable, arbitrary, or capricious. Appellees, as found by the Board, were guilty of dishonorable and unprofessional conduct and the licenses issued to the appellees by the Board should be revoked. We hold that the trial judge substituted his judgement for the the judgement of the Board; therefore, the decision of the trial court is reversed and the case remanded with instructions to affirm the decision of the Board." (Seidenberg v. New Mexico Board of Medical Examiners, 1969).

Why are boards of medical examiners not more adept at avoiding legal pitfalls? The answer in most cases is not lack of legal counsel but lack of continuity of advice. In many states the attorney for the board is assigned by the attorney general. Often he is a junior member of the staff and the board might have different counsel at each meeting. It is not unusual for a strange attorney to be summoned to a board meeting on short notice with no opportunity to familiarize himself with the law or policies of the board. Lucky is the board which, by law, is permitted to retain its own legal counsel. A competent lawyer can soon become an expert in the handling of licensing matters and can turn out to be of great assistance to the board. While his viewpoint might differ from that of the board members, in that he is more interested in the coldly legalistic aspects of discipline than in the personal problems of physicians, this is a healthy situation as it provides balance. His job is to instruct the board members in the law, thereby helping them to follow proper procedures and arrive at just verdicts that cannot be successfully challenged in the courts.

Purposely I have all but ignored the 71 per cent of the cases in which the boards of medical examiners have been upheld by the courts. This is because an analysis of failures is more instructive than dwelling upon successes. The fact that in the majority of instances the courts do uphold the boards indicates that their actions are usually not hasty and ill advised. Despite the loud accusations of their detractors, the boards on the whole are doing a good job in the difficult field of medical discipline. Their performance will be improved when obvious flaws in their medical practice laws are eliminated by proper amendments.

Bibliography

American Medical Association. 1967. *Disciplinary Digest:* Chicago.
———. 1967. *The Citation.* 17:2. (Supplement).
Board of Medical Examiners v. *Schutzbank.* 94 Ariz. 281, 383 P. 2d 192 (1963).

CHAPTER EIGHT

THE MEDICAL IMPOSTOR

This is a true story. Freddie Brant was born 43 years ago in Louisiana. Reared in poverty, his formal education ended with the fifth grade. During World War II he was in the army for four years. After discharge he found that jobs were scarce for a man with only a fifth-grade education; therefore he joined the paratroops. In 1949, along with a fellow paratrooper he was sentenced to seven years in the penitentiary for bank robbery. There he worked in the prison hospital, thus beginning his medical education. Finally released, he obtained his postgraduate medical education by working as a laboratory and X-ray technician for Dr. Reid L. Brown of Chattanooga, Tennessee. This job lasted for four years during which he picked up more medical lore, along with the diplomas of his employer.

He was now ready to begin the practice of medicine. Assuming the identity of Dr. Reid L. Brown, he moved to Texas where he obtained a license by endorsement and served for three years on the staff of the State Hospital at Terrell. He then resigned and took his wife on a vacation trip. Stopping in the small village of Groveton, Texas for a Coca Cola, he treated the injured leg of a child. He found that Groveton had long been without a doctor and the people were clamoring for medical care. "Dr. Brown" soon became established as the town physician and as a community leader.

Freddie Brant, alias Reid L. Brown, M.D., might still be carrying on his thriving practice in Groveton, Texas, had he not run afoul of the computer. By coincidence he ordered drugs from the same pharmaceutical firm in New Orleans patronized by the real Dr. Reid Brown. The computer gagged when it discovered orders on the same day from physicians with identical names in Groveton and Chattanooga. Following an investigation, Freddie Brant was charged with forgery and with false testimony that he was a doctor.

The exposure of Freddie Brant caused consternation in Groveton. But the citizens rallied around their "doctor"; many were the testimonials to his skill. According to one news report, the list of his patients included some of the leading citizens, as well as farmers, loggers, and welfare patients. The druggist said that many cases of hardship were caused by the arrest of Freddie. A particularly glowing testimonial came from a farmer who said, "My wife has been sick for 14 years. We've been to doctors in Lufkin, Crockett, and Trinity and he did her more good than any of 'em. She was all drawed up, bent over, you ought to have seen her. He's brought her up and now she's milking cows and everything."

The citizens of Groveton remained loyal to Brant. A grand jury refused to indict him. Authorities then brought him to trial in another county for perjury but the case ended in a hung jury with eight members for acquittal. According to *Chicago's American* (July 26, 1968), justice was thwarted because of a "lava flow of testimonials from Groveton and Terrell to the effect that Freddie Brant was a prince of a medical man, license or no license." In an unkind cut, the same paper said that the people of Groveton should have known that Reid Brown was not a doctor as he did too many things wrong. For example, he made house calls for five dollars and charged only three dollars for an office call; he approved of Medicare and would drive for miles to visit a patient, often without fee if the person were poor; besides, his handwriting was legible.

What were the secrets of Freddie Brant's success as an impersonator? They were many, but the main ones were his readiness to refer any potentially complicated cases to nearby towns, a personality which inspired confidence, and a willingness to take time to listen to his patients.

Freddie Brant is only one of many medical impostors whose records are on file in the Department of Investigation of the American Medical Association. My study of medical impostors is based both upon my own experience and an analysis of the records of the Department of Investigation. However, this wealth of material does not lend itself to statistical analysis. Consequently, my conclusions will be based upon some general observations as well as selected case histories. I attempted to find the answers to several questions, such as the medical background of the impostors, their routes to practice, the number who had diplomas or licenses, real or forged, the length of time that their hoaxes were successful, their manner of exposure, and the reactions of the public to them after their exposure.

Let us take a look at the typical successful impostor. His medical background might consist of a tour of duty as a medical corpsman in the Army or as a pharmacist's mate in the Navy. He might have served as a hospital orderly or as a laboratory technician. Some obtain their medical educations as patients in mental hospitals. The sole medical background of one was service as an elevator operator in a hospital. From his associations with physicians the impostor acquires a smattering of medical jargon sufficient to fool the unwary. But our impostor must have other attributes in addition to facility in enlarging his vocabulary; the most important of these are a good memory and a persuasive manner.

State hospitals, particularly in recent years, have provided an entree into fraudulent medical practice. I found six such cases in the last ten years. One of the most interesting is that of a person without medical background who was employed as superintendent of a state hospital. His credentials were based solely upon a diploma stolen from a Dr. Menendez, a graduate of the University of Havana Medical School. This man might have enjoyed a long and profitable career as a hospital administrator. But he resigned after nine months and moved to another region where he obtained a position as staff psychiatrist in a state hospital mainly on the basis of his recommendations from the first state. However, his second career was cut short when his new colleagues became suspicious because of his manner and exposed him. Obviously he committed a grave error by resigning his high position as a hospital superintendent. I could not learn his reasons for doing so; possibly he became tired of administrative duties and yearned to return to clinical psychiatry.

Whatever mild amusement I derived from the story of "Dr. Menendez" soon turned to dismay as I read on. The director of the Department of Health in the state in which he was first employed, whose duty it was to pass upon the credentials of this impostor, said that the state hospital was hiring some recognized foreign doctors on a temporary basis. Obviously his examination of these credentials was entirely superficial.

While the authorities in neither state should have been taken in by "Dr. Menendez," there might be extenuating circumstances, all too familiar to members of boards of medical examiners. First, there is a concerted effort among certain groups in the United States to resettle foreign physicians, particularly those who are thought to be fugitives from communism; secondly, there is a universal shortage of qualified applicants for staff positions in state hospitals so that the standards are deliberately lowered to permit physicians unqualified for regular licenses to fill them. Thirdly, highly placed politicians often intercede for them. These three factors combine to place such pressure on boards of medical examiners that it is remarkable that they resist as effectively as they do.

There are other reasons why state hospitals offer such good opportunities for fraudulent practice. In many states applicants for positions are not required to be screened by the boards of medical examiners. Where licenses are not required, special permits to practice only in the hospital are granted. Some states have no requirements. Where the hospital authorities are the sole judges of credentials, they have neither the facilities nor the inclination to carry out adequate investigations.

How long do impostors flourish? The files of the Department of Investigation contain the records of at least 15 impostors who practiced successfully for over a year. There were two whose hoaxes lasted for 20 years. Perhaps the all-time champion was "Dr. J. D. Phillips" who practiced medicine in various places for 30 years. According to an article in *Coronet* (August, 1953) he fooled not only patients in 11 states but also the United States government, several county and state health departments, and dozens of respectable physicians, nurses, and administrators in various hospitals. Said *Coronet*, "Rarely has a faker been unmasked more often and less permanently. Certainly no one has gone to so much trouble to remain loyal to his profession." His medical knowledge was gained from the doctor in his home town with whom he made rounds. Said "Dr. Phillips" without undue modesty, "So I went around with him and absorbed it all. I have a photographic memory and I am not exactly dumb."

"Dr. Phillips" served time in various penitentiaries for passing bad checks and for defrauding hotels. He used these periods to study in the prison libraries. Finally his background was so firm that he was entrusted with surgery at the Maryland State House of Correction. According to the physician in charge, he was "literally a good resident." At some time during this period he was able to steal a medical license from a physician long inactive because of illness. He then had the temerity to send an affidavit to his adopted alma mater that he had lost his M.D. diploma. He was promptly furnished with a duplicate.

"Dr. Phillips's" downfall was finally brought about by his greed and an alert insurance agent. He was involved in an automobile accident in which he suffered injuries to his neck and arm. He was sued for $600. He countered with a $40,000 suit, demanding $35,000 to compensate him for his inability to practice medicine. The insurance agent, disturbed by his dirty fingernails, questioned his story and he was exposed in court. His medical career is now at an end as he was sentenced to 15 to 20 years for perjury.

How are impostors exposed? Obviously those whose medical careers last only a few months are so inept that they give themselves away. But exposure of the experts has proven difficult and frequently happens only by accident. Several have allowed their greed to get the better of them and have tried to supplement their incomes from medical practice by various confidence games. As far as I know, Freddie Brant is the only one who has been exposed by the computer.

A surprising discovery was the fact that few impostors had credentials either in the form of medical school diplomas or state medical licenses. Detailed examination of the records of 30 successful impostors revealed that only eight had bothered to obtain credentials either by forgery or theft. Such oversight is amazing. I found that there is a firm in California which specializes in producing phony documents. At least one impostor was familiar with this company; he not only ordered complete medical credentials but also turned himself into an author. He removed the pages from a book and had them rebound with his name on the cover. His fatal mistake was in failing to realize that he might be called upon by a colleague to discuss the contents.

The attitude of some impostors seems to be, why bother to obtain phony diplomas when they are not necessary? I am astonished at the number of hospitals which have accepted applicants for positions without first examining their credentials. This is not confined to state hospitals. A glaring example is the recent case of "Dr. David William Baker" who claimed to have graduated from Temple University Medical School in 1962. From a state hospital in Idaho he went to Seattle where he worked in two hospitals for a total of three months. For two months he worked in the emergency room of one hospital. According to a Seattle newspaper, a hospital spokesman said that Baker had been hired on the recommendation of a doctor who had known him when he worked at the blood bank. The hospital only detected the imposture when it learned that the American Medical Association had sent out a circular saying that a man named Baker was posing as a doctor. The justification of the administrator: Baker claimed his credentials were in transit and he was preparing to appear before the state licensing board. Hospital officials weakly contended that he was not a member of the staff but worked in the emergency room where he was always under the supervision of another physician.

The gullibility of the public, both medical and non-medical, struck me. I was astonished by the readiness of bankers, whom I had always regarded as paragons of caution, to lend money to impostors to help them start their medical practices. In one instance a physician was the victim when he lent an impostor a considerable sum of money. Also fair game are the citizens of many small towns with desperate shortages of doctors who will lionize any presentable individual who claims to be a physician.

Granted that the charm and persuasive powers of the successful quack in any field are considerable; however, I am amazed at the failure of responsible citizens to question his credentials.

Another curious phenomenon is the reaction of the public after the exposure of the impostor. Many people staunchly defend him and are grievously hurt because the authorities have removed their trusted family physician. Typical is the case of the fraud who, for some six years, successfully practiced in a small town in New York State. His following of devoted patients was large. He even won the esteem of his colleagues who frequently called upon him for consultations. When he was finally exposed by the agents of the State Board of Medical Examiners, the anguished outcries of his devoted followers could be heard all the way across the Hudson River. They even circulated petitions to prevent him from being banished. Nevertheless he was brought to justice and convicted of fraud.

The reactions of these people and of those in Groveton, Texas, to the unmasking of Freddie Brant are by no means isolated examples. This attitude is particularly prevalent in small towns. One can only speculate as to why these victims of hoaxes adopt such defensive attitudes. Possibly they feel that they must justify their faith in the impostor to avoid the appearance of stupidity in the eyes of their neighbors. Or, in some instances, they may be compared with the victim of any confidence game who refuses to report the operator because of his own personal embarrassment.

Another difficulty in exposing medical impostors stems from the indifference of the district attorneys. I have had personal experience with this and from my conversations with other members of boards of medical examiners I have learned that my problem is not unique. Apparently these law enforcers are not enthusiastic about pursuing people whom they regard as petty criminals, for this is just what they are in many states. In only four states, Florida, Kentucky, New Mexico, and Rhode Island, is the practice of medicine without a license defined as a felony. In the other 46 it is a misdemeanor. I remember one instance in which my board of medical examiners discovered a man who was practicing medicine without a license. On two different occasions the investigator for the board obtained receipted bills, copies of prescriptions, and samples of drugs the man had been dispensing, certainly more than sufficient evidence for the conviction of this fraud. But the district attorney showed no interest in prosecuting him. It was not until some two years later, after the impostor had been responsible for the death of a patient, that the state police arrested him on a charge of manslaughter for which he was convicted and sentenced to five years in prison.

The attitude of the newspapers towards some impostors is interesting. While they make every effort to report the facts accurately, in their stories there is sometimes a strong underlying note of amusement. In the case just cited, after the impostor had been arrested and charged with manslaughter, the local paper printed a feature article in its Sunday edition based upon an interview in the jail cell of the felon. This took the form of a human interest story which depicted the impostor as an amusing eccentric and all but ignored the charge of manslaughter.

Up to a point, many of the tales of impersonation *are* amusing, provided the reader is not one of the authorities who has been duped; but the time must come when one has to be serious, particularly when one thinks of the danger that impostors pose to the public. Freddie Brant, alias "Dr. Brown," the Texas impersonator, tried to justify his conduct by saying, "I never lost a patient." Didn't he? How can he know? Another famous impostor, M. L. Langford of Jasper, Missouri, pointed out in his defense that he performed no surgery and referred any patient who might have complications. But could he always recognize complications or foresee them? Impostors *do* kill people, albeit not always as dramatically as the notorious Dr. Frank who was implicated in five deaths in Chicago. He was a former mental patient who persuaded a physician to help him obtain a listing with a medical referring service. He then took over the practice of a vacationing doctor. (See *Chicago Tribune*, December 3, 1958.)

A natural question is, what motivates these people to impersonate doctors? The immediate answer of the cynic is that they do it to make money. While it is true that some yearn for the imagined rich and easy life of the doctor, this is not the only answer. Some envy the authority and social position of the doctor. Others are mentally deranged, many having served terms in mental hospitals. Freddie Brant simply said, "I always wanted to be a doctor."

Up to this point I have confined my discussion to the modus operandi of medical impostors. I must now inquire into how they can be controlled. Obviously, as in disease, the best cure is prevention. Today several agencies are responsible for the proper screening of physicians. The most important of these are the boards of medical examiners, the medical societies, and the hospitals. It should be primarily the duty of the boards of medical examiners to see that all who seek to practice medicine in their states are qualified. More careful screening of applicants for positions in state hospitals should be carried out, preferably by the licensing boards. The boards must ascertain that all applicants are the possessors of the credentials submitted and they cannot accept them on faith; they must investigate them at their sources no matter how impeccable the appearance of the applicant. Their investigations should be systematic, beginning with insistence upon completion of a detailed application blank which must provide space for a notarized statement from the applicant that he is indeed the person whose credentials he is presenting. It is important that the physician be required to present at least two photographs, one to be affixed to the form, the other to be filed for future reference in case of a question of identity. As an added precaution the board might insist that the photograph be affixed to the application form before it is returned to the medical school for certification or, in the case of licensure by endorsement, to the board issuing the original license.

Another important method of preventing licensure of impostors is the use of the personal interview. In states which license large numbers of physicians it might be difficult for the administrative officer to interview all of them. In these states the interview could be divided up among the members of the board. Although opinions differ in regard to the value of the interview, an experienced person should be able to learn much by observing a candidate. He can train himself to recognize certain danger signals such as poor personal grooming, vague answers to specific questions concerning medical subjects, and failure to identify properly professors in the school from which the applicant claims to have graduated.

Still another method of detecting impostors is the requirement that all applicants for licensure be fingerprinted. Many boards of medical examiners are reluctant to require this as they feel that the professional man should not be embarrassed by such an indignity. At present only seven boards require fingerprinting. But this is not as drastic a requirement as many think and most applicants submit to it with good grace. After all, fingerprinting is required in applications for many jobs, particularly those associated with the federal government. An interesting observation was made by Sprecher (1968) regarding fingerprinting of applicants for the bar. He found that the mere requirement will encourage applicants to admit to previous convictions of crimes. For example, bar examinations were given in Michigan and Illinois at the same time. Michigan had 281 applicants, Illinois, 273. Both states asked the question, "Have you ever been charged with a crime or arrested?" In Michigan, where fingerprinting is required, 28 people, or 10 per cent, admitted to previous arrests or convictions. In Illinois, which did not require fingerprinting, only two, or less than one per cent, made such admissions.

If the practice of medicine without a license were a felony instead of a misdemeanor, as it is in most states, some impostors might be deterred.

Finally, how can impostors be detected after they have established their practices as physicians? Without a doubt the most authoritative source of information concerning physicians is the Department of Investigation of the American Medical Association. In its files are kept the complete biographical records of all physicians from the time they first enter medical school until they die. If they drop out of school, this also is noted. After graduation, up-to-date records are kept of internships, residencies, types and places of practice, and of any difficulties physicians might have with the law, their boards of medical examiners and medical societies. Records of graduates of foreign medical schools who come to this country are also kept. Furthermore, the Department of Investigation is able to conduct a complete search at the request of a hospital, board of medical examiners, or a medical society to determine whether or not a person really is a physician. A typical investigation involves reference to the active file, the new name file, the AMA directory, the medical student dropout file, in addition to a meticulous examination of at least nine directories. If the suspect's name cannot be found by such an exhaustive investigation, one can be certain that he is not a doctor, and many is the impostor who has been brought to light on the basis of a search by the Department of Investigation.

According to H. Doyle Taylor,* director of the Department of Investigation, the Department was created in 1906 as the brain child of the late Arthur Cramp, M.D. As associate editor of the *Journal of the American Medical Association*, he had launched a campaign for reform in advertising of patent medicines. At first most of the inquiries directed to the department came from physicians who wanted information concerning the blatantly advertised nostrums promising cure of every disease from diabetes, tuberculosis, and venereal disease to diphtheria. Although these nostrums have been eliminated through government regulations, the quacks have adapted to the times and now find ready markets among the gullible public for baldness cures, cancer cures, breast de-

* Personal communication.

velopers, worthless vitamins, and insomnia treatments, to list a few of their "cures."

During recent years the Department of Investigation has concentrated its efforts on health education of the public through the circulation of literature, exhibits, and films in an effort to create better understanding of quackery and its evils. Today most of the thousands of inquiries received every year come from the public.

The Department of Investigation works closely with the Food and Drug Administration, the Post Office Department, the Federal Trade Commission, the American Cancer Society and many other public and private agencies, including law enforcement officers, in its unremitting war against quackery. In addition, its staff of 11 people has catalogued the most extensive files available on the subject and constantly keeps them up to date. The Department played prominent parts in the "Krebiozen" trial involving the controversial cancer treatment and also in exposure of the notorious "Dr. Hoxsey," and his fake cancer remedy. Furthermore, many fraudulent schemes are now being exposed before they become firmly entrenched. For instance, the Department of Investigation, working with the Ohio State Medical Society and the Cleveland Academy of Medicine, stopped distribution of the worthless Rand cancer vaccine before it had a chance to create false hopes for too many victims.

The guiding spirits of the Department of Investigation, Director H. Doyle Taylor and Research Director Oliver Field, as well as all of the other members of the staff burn with a missionary zeal and are quick to respond to any request for an investigation of a suspected fraud. Although lacking in legal authority, they have helped to convict many charlatans and impostors by their willingness to provide expert testimony in court.

In the past, the advantages of the Department of Investigation have not been fully appreciated. But in May 1968, mainly with the cooperation of the American Hospital Association, it widely circulated information concerning its available services. The results immediately became apparent; in May

1968 the Department was asked to screen routinely a total of 1,139 applicants for licensure, hospital staff appointments and membership in medical societies. In June it received 3,885 such requests, more than a threefold increase, and the number continues to grow.

If responsible agencies such as boards of medical examiners, hospital staffs, and medical societies take all possible precautions, only rarely will a medical impostor slip by them. But no system can be infallible, and, because of man's never-ending quest for a state of complete physical well being, the occasional glib charlatan, once he evades the authorities, is likely to survive. In this event it is the job of all concerned to make his survival time as short as possible.

Bibliography

Chicago's American, July 26, 1968.
Coronet, August 1953.
Sprecher, Robert. 1968. Licensure Problems in the Legal Profession. *Fed. Bull.* 55:188–200.

CHAPTER NINE

BASIC SCIENCE LAWS

A curious phenomenon of medical licensure is the gradual proliferation and the persistence of basic science laws. Since the enactment of the first law by Wisconsin in 1925, the legislatures of 24 states have passed them.* Originally they were designed to test the competence in the basic sciences of all members of the "healing arts," but now there are so many exceptions that the only practitioners required to have basic science certificates are M.D.'s, osteopaths, chiropractors, and in certain states, naturopaths.

All of the states which finally adopted basic science laws generally patterned them after the original law of Wisconsin. This statute provided for the establishment of a separate board of examiners in the basic sciences to examine all candidates for licensure by the various boards of the healing arts. Before an individual could be considered for licensure he was required to possess a certificate of proficiency in the basic sciences. Only then could he be licensed to practice by the appropriate board. The basic science certificate is just that and not a license to practice.

Today medical educators and physicians alike are becoming increasingly exasperated with the additional barriers to licensure which the basic science laws present. In these days of rapid growth of medical knowledge, the burgeoning of medical education, and the increasing mobility of the population, basic science requirements are considered by many to be anachronistic stumbling blocks to medical licensure. In addition they cause waste of time and financial hardship particularly to the

* The District of Columbia also has a basic science law. For the purposes of this discussion it is considered a state.

impecunious resident who frequently must make an extra trip to a distant state to take a basic science examination.

To learn the reasons for the adoption of basic science laws by 24 states one must inquire into the history of the movement in Wisconsin. According to Taylor (1931), the medical practice acts were not protecting the public against quackery except in the medical profession. Often the legal definition of the practice of medicine was not sufficiently broad; as a result, the activities of cultists fell outside the definition and were repeatedly found proper in court, thanks to clever and unscrupulous lawyers. Taylor said, "We found that while our own medical practice act was intended not only to elevate the standards of medical practice but also to protect the public against all quacks, actually it was serving only to maintain a high standard for physicians."

The Medical Society of Wisconsin believed that passage of a basic science law would assure the public that all who treated the sick would at least be qualified to exercise care and skill in making a diagnosis.

Taylor stated that before the passage of the Wisconsin law 200 uneducated healers were coming into the state each year and practicing despite the apparent safeguards of public health legislation. Five and a half years later, after the passage of the basic science law, he asserted that there was none who lasted beyond the first call of the investigator of the board. However, he gave no source for his figures.

Incidentally, Tennessee antedated Wisconsin in the application of the basic science principle. According to Woodward (1929), in 1915 the legislature created a Board of Preliminary Examiners and provided for preliminary examinations in the basic sciences. Woodward also thought that the laws regulating the practice of medicine were not accomplishing their purpose, and that, while they insured the competence of practitioners of medicine, the good accomplished had been offset by the legalization and entrenchment of many cults.

He summed up the philosophy of the champions of basic science laws as follows: "The reasonableness of the plan outlined is obvious. It recognizes that a certain knowledge of anatomy, physiology, pathology and diagnosis is at the basis of all diagnosis and treatment whatever. It recognizes that the possession of such knowledge by all practitioners is necessary for the safety of the public. It ignores all differences of opinion among practitioners as to the methods of diagnosis and treatment and sets up a nonprofessional board, representing the public, to determine the fundamental fitness of all would-be practitioners. Such candidates as this nonsectarian board has determined to be fit, and no others, are permitted to appear before the professional examining boards."

The original Wisconsin Basic Science Board, composed of three members, none of whom could belong to any branch of the healing arts, included two biologists and a chemist (Guyer, 1926). Granted that the law provided that the board members were permitted to seek consultation in devising examinations, the fact remains that the evaluation of competence to practice the healing arts was in the hands of nonmembers. Apparently the authors of the law considered this a master stroke because the board could not be accused of partiality to any one branch.

The passage of the basic science law in Wisconsin was not easy and required several attempts because of the united opposition of the osteopaths, chiropractors, and other cultists. But finally the state medical society was able to hail it as a signal victory.

Only a few weeks after the enactment of the law by the Wisconsin legislature a basic science law was passed in Connecticut. This was an emergency action to deal with a crisis brought on by the influx of graduates of diploma mills.

The following table shows the years in which the various states enacted basic science laws. There certainly was no rush to adopt them as evidenced by the long period encompassed and the fact that no more than three states passed them in any one year.

The efficacy of the basic science system was soon challenged by Bierring. In an editorial (Federation of State Medical Boards, 1928) he stated that he had found several inconsistencies in the basic science acts. While candidates for medical licensure must present evidence of having completed a pre-

Table 7.   Years of Enactment of Basic Science Laws[a]

1925	–	Connecticut, Wisconsin
1927	–	Minnesota, Nebraska, Washington
1929	–	District of Columbia
1934	–	Oregon
1935	–	Iowa, Tennessee
1936	–	Arizona
1937	–	Colorado, Michigan, Oklahoma
1939	–	Florida, South Dakota
1940	–	Rhode Island
1941	–	New Mexico
1945	–	Alaska
1949	–	Texas
1951	–	Nevada
1957	–	Kansas
1959	–	Arkansas, Utah (became effective in 1961)
1960	–	Alabama

[a] From *J.A.M.A.* 180:892 (1962).

scribed course of study in prescribed subjects, the candidates appearing before the basic science boards were not required to have any such qualifications. "A graduate of a chiropractic school who has not seen the inside of a laboratory of chemistry, pathology or bacteriology is permitted the same privileges as the graduates of some of our leading medical institutions." He concluded that the basic science laws were of distinct advantage to the cultist but did not further higher standards of medical licensure.

In 1930 Bierring gave qualified support to the basic science movement when he stated that from the information at hand it appeared that the purposes of the basic science laws had been accomplished. But he pointed to certain flaws in the statutes such as undue emphasis on the examination as the sole test of knowledge without regard to the quality of previous training. He also called attention to the disagreement as to what subjects constituted the basic sciences even in the original six laws. He objected to the lack of uniformity of personnel composing the boards. He injected a note of caution, subsequently ignored, that the basic science boards should be given proper discretion so that graduates of approved medical schools who had been more than adequately tested in the basic sciences might be excused from an extra examination.

The supporters of basic science laws became enthusiastic in their praise of them. For example, in 1938 DuBois of Minnesota proclaimed that the laws insured better trained men for every branch of the "healing arts." He wrote, "Perhaps not better trained medical men, as Minnesota accepts only products of approved medical schools, but surely better trained cultists." And I add, pray tell me what is a well-trained cultist? And what use do cultists make of training in the basic sciences other than to memorize enough facts to pass an examination?

In 1943, when only 17 states had basic science laws, Clements emphasized the good in them despite their diversity. He then, paradoxically, pointed to the great variation in qualifications of board members, the lack of uniformity of the laws in subjects required, methods of examination and passing grades, all of which caused difficulty in reciprocity. He said, "While due caution in the matter of waiver may entail some inconvenience for some bona fide candidates, this is far out-weighed by the common good sought. The best evidence in support of the basic science laws is that the boards are generally regarded as functioning well and that other states are trying to get such laws."

However, Clements based his arguments upon generalities and after he made this statement only seven more states enacted basic science laws.

Madison (1947) proposed uniform laws, emphasizing the necessity for standardization of subjects, type, and length of examinations and passing grades so that they could be adjudged equivalent by the legal authorities when the boards sought reciprocity. Although he was optimistic in believing that standard basic science laws would be adopted, he described the absurdity of the laws of his own state of Michigan which could also be applied to other states. He referred to the number of subjects a candidate is allowed to fail before he is required to repeat the whole examination. Unlike the system in colleges where the student must repeat the examinations only in the subjects in which he was deficient, in the basic science examinations, if he fails two subjects he has to repeat all of them. On the next try he might fail two other subjects but pass the ones he failed on the first examination. Again, he must repeat the whole examination. "The logical question is, when does a student pass an individual subject? He passes the subject once and fails it the next time; so when has he passed it? It would be funny if it were not so tragic." The same absurd situation can apply to some medical examinations.

Platter (1946), for many years secretary of the Ohio medical board, was an implacable foe of basic science laws. He could see no reason why graduates of approved medical schools should be required to take basic science examinations. Furthermore, he stated that these laws do not prevent the illegal practice of medicine despite the contention of their advocates that the laws are self-enforcing and their inference that it would be impossible for an individual to practice any form of the healing arts without a basic science certificate.

Crowe (1942), another enemy of basic science laws, called them hurdles in the pathways of some of the world's most competent physicians. He said that the laws sounded good but they failed to establish a single high standard of practice. He objected to the failure to include diagnosis as the major subject of examinations. "No doctor can protect the public against a disease he cannot recognize, the existence of which he may even doubt, as do those who scoff at the idea of infectious organisms and insist that all human ills are the result of an anatomic deviation or defect."

In 1941 Carter defended basic science laws with the unanswerable assertion that no state, having passed one, had repealed it. On the other hand, he conceded that unqualified people could pass the examinations by drills in questions and answers. He referred to certain cram courses which were available to the ignorant candidates.

Madison (1943), in calling attention to the difficulties in endorsement and reciprocity, said that comparison of the laws indicated that it was nearly impossible for any states to have reciprocity with each other. Yet boards had entered into reciprocity relations in direct violation of the laws which created them. The difficulties were due to the wide variations in the laws and in the policies of the boards. He said, "The present state of heterogeneity in basic science and practices, each aiming at the same goal, yet hindering each other more than helping in the attainment of their goal, points to a need for some kind of unified command for our activities. This might take the form of some kind of a national organization of state basic science boards." Such an organization was later established, but it has done little to correct the situation.

After the last basic science law was passed in Alabama in 1960 criticism of the laws became unfashionable for a time. In fact, in certain circles, even questioning of the effectiveness of the laws was viewed with dismay and considered equal to an attack upon the Holy Trinity. In 1961 I introduced a resolution at the meeting of the Federation of State Medical Boards of the United States that the organization recommend the abolishment of the basic science laws. This brought forth long and acrimonious discussion and passage of a motion to table; this, despite the fact that for many years one of the chief aims of the Federation had been the promotion of interstate endorsement and reciprocity. One of the clinching arguments was that the basic science boards were outside the province of the Federation and, therefore, should not be criticized. (See Minutes in Federation of State Medical Boards, 1961.) By the conclusion of the argument I was made to feel as if I had attacked a basic American institution such as wedded motherhood or the flag.

In 1963 the Federation, at its annual meeting, conducted a panel discussion on the subject, "Obstacles to Universal Reciprocity and Endorsement." Of necessity the basic science laws were considered. I was asked to discuss this aspect of the problem and as background I presented the results of a survey based on questionnaires sent to the secretaries of the boards of medical examiners (Derbyshire, 1963). Cooperation was perfect; replies were received from all 50 states and the District of Columbia. Two sets of questions were sent out, one to the states not having basic science laws and a different one to those which did have them. At that time 24 states, including the District of Columbia, had basic science laws. The questionnaire (below) shows the opinions of the secretaries of the medical boards of non-basic science states. Noteworthy was the fact that not one considered that a basic science law would be of any value in his state. A large majority thought that the laws did not prevent quacks and cultists from flourishing, and a majority believed that basic science laws interfered with reciprocity and endorsement.

Opinions of secretaries of medical boards having no basic science laws[a]

1. Has your legislature ever seriously considered passing a Basic Science Law? (No–25; Yes–2.)

2. If so, who sponsored it? (In both instances the State Medical Society and in both states it was lost in a committee of the legislature. One secretary specifically stated that it was opposed by osteopaths, chiropractors and others.)

3. If a Basic Science Law has been introduced and defeated, why, and who opposed it? (This question proved to be unnecessary in view of the answers included under 2.)

4. Do you believe that a Basic Science Law now would be advantageous in your state? (No–27; Yes–0.)

5. Does the lack of a Basic Science Law now permit quacks and cultists to flourish? (No–25; Yes–2.)

6. Do you believe that Basic Science Laws hinder reciprocity among the state boards of medical examiners? (Yes–21; No–3; No opinion–3.)

The second questionnaire shows the results of an inquiry directed to the secretaries of boards whose states had basic science laws. These states seemed, on the whole, to think that the laws were accomplishing their purpose, although they were not always sure as to what this was. Basic science laws are not confined to any one region but can be found from the New England states to the Pacific coast. Of questionable significance is the fact that of the 24 states which had passed the laws, 18 were located west of the Mississippi River.

[a] From Derbyshire, 1963.

Opinions of secretaries of medical boards having basic science laws

1. When was your Basic Science Law passed? (The first was passed in Wisconsin in 1925, the most recent in Utah in 1961. The dates of adoption are well scattered throughout the years and it is evident that in no one year or period was there a rush by the states to adopt these laws.)

2. What is the personnel of your board and how is it appointed? (Practically all of the boards are appointed by the governors of the states. Concerning the personnel of the boards there is much variation: Not specified but no M.D.'s–5; M.D.'s and osteopaths–2; M.D.'s, chiropractors, osteopaths, and "others"–4; two members of faculties of colleges and one pathologist–1; members can have no connection with the healing arts–8; M.D.'s only–3.)

3. Who is responsible for the passage of your Basic Science Law? (The State Medical Society–20; Board of Medical Examiners–5; Osteopaths–2; Public Health Department–2; General Public–2. In some cases the replies indicated that more than one agency was responsible, hence the discrepancy in the figures.)

4. Who first thought that a Basic Science Law was necessary? (State Medical Society–12; Health Department–1; Public–1; Board of Medical Examiners–1; Do not know–8.)

5. When the law was passed, what was it supposed to accomplish? (Prevent licensing of unqualified persons–15; Keep out chiropractors and osteopaths–1; Keep out osteopaths, chiropractors and naturopaths–2; Control chiropractors–3; Do not know–1; To keep out a particular group–1.)

6. Has it accomplished its purpose? (Yes–15; No–6; Partially–1; Unable to state–1.)

7. If the answer to the above is no, in what respects has it failed? (Of course, there were individual remarks in reply to this but in general they may be classified as follows: It has discouraged M.D.'s from settling in the state but has not kept out undesirable people–4; It has not kept out any undesirable groups–2; Due to a flaw in the statute it is worthless–1.)

8. Do you believe that the Basic Science requirement has tended to discourage well-qualified doctors of medicine from settling in your state? (No–16; Yes–7.)

9. Do you believe that the reciprocity policies of your Basic Science Board are sufficiently liberal? (Yes–20; No–3.)

10. Do you believe that the Basic Science Law has prevented cultists and quacks from flourishing? (Yes–14; Yes, to a limited extent–4; No–5.)

11. Do you think your Basic Science Law should be repealed? (No–18; Yes–5.)

12. Does your Basic Science Law interfere in any respect with reciprocity agreements with other states insofar as licenses to practice medicine are concerned? (No–13; Yes–10.)

13. Are the meetings of the Basic Science Board and of the Board of Medical Examiners coordinated so that undue delay in issuing licenses on the basis of examinations does not occur? (Yes–19; No–2; Unknown–2.)

At first glance there was apparently universal agreement among the states not having basic science laws. All seemed to believe that they were undesirable, that they accomplished no useful purpose, and that they had failed to attain their original goals. The problem among those states could have been disposed of simply had I been able to disregard one disquieting factor, namely that in one state as recently as 1961 a basic science law went into effect, even though the president of the board of medical examiners viewed it with distaste. I wondered at the time whether or not the trend towards such legislation would continue and which of the remaining 27 states would be the next to succumb. So far there have been no others.

The lack of uniformity of the basic science laws noted by earlier authors was found to continue. If one considers that the composition of the boards varies from no M.D.'s at all to all M.D.'s and from a mixture of M.D.'s, osteopaths and chiropractors to complete exclusion of anyone connected with the healing arts, one can only conclude that the laws represent a patchwork dictated by various political compromises. The policies of the various boards are capricious and vary from month to month. For example, I know of one candidate for endorsement of his basic science certificate who, when he took his examinations in the first state, was delayed by a sleet storm so that he missed the examination in one subject. He passed all of the other examinations and at the next meeting of the board also passed the one he had missed; but the other state would not accept his certificate because it had a rule that all of the examinations had to be taken at one sitting. Consequently he had to repeat the examinations in the second state at great cost and inconvenience.

Important is the fact that the state medical societies were responsible for the passage of basic science laws. I cannot deny that their motives were lofty despite the often heard accusations that the doctors wanted to keep out competition. Organized medicine should be proud that legislatures will usually heed its recommendations if they believe that such recommendations contribute to the health and safety of the public. But how many of the members of state medical societies who strove so mightily for the passage of these laws now regret their actions? Or how many even understand them? The question is difficult to answer and I can only cite one of our senior citizens in the profession who, when pointing with pride to his accomplishments, placed the passage of the basic science law high on his list. When asked what it had accomplished and why it should not be repealed, he quickly changed the subject!

The possible effectiveness of the laws has been negated by the fact that many cultists can pass the examinations even though several attempts are sometimes necessary. Several secretaries of medical boards stated that the examinations were directed at one or two particular groups. Therefore, it is inconceivable that the laws truly contribute to the public health and safety since they require qualified doctors of medicine to negotiate an extra, expensive, time consuming hurdle on the way to licensure in an attempt to exclude a few chiropractors, many of whom can pass the examinations, anyway.

As did earlier authors, I found many inconsistencies concerning the proper subjects for examination. It is remarkable that after almost 40 years the states are still unable to agree on the subjects of the basic sciences. Some states require examinations in hygiene or public health, while other boards examine the candidates in subjects supposedly at the college level, although even superficial inspection of the questions will convince one that they should have attended medical school for at least two years before attempting to pass the examinations.

There is a hodgepodge of grandfather clauses running through the laws which will permit an individual to receive a certificate without examination if he has been in practice a certain number of years. For example, in one state a candidate who has been in practice for 19 years must prove that he is learned in the basic sciences by passing an examination, whereas one year later he can receive a certificate by waiver. Does this mean that after 20 years of practice a physician has no need for proficiency in the basic sciences? Does the passage of a year automatically endow him with the necessary knowledge? Or is it possible that such a rule is based upon political expediency?

One glaring inconsistency was found in the law of one state which excuses candidates from taking the basic science examinations if they had had service in World War II or if they were in school in 1939. This represents the epitome of irrelevance and must have been brought about by some devious political compromise.

In 1964 I entered the lion's den when I addressed the American Association of Basic Science Boards on the subject, "Should There Be Basic Science Boards?" (See Derbyshire, 1965.) In preparing this address, I broadened the original survey to include attorneys general of the states, the boards of osteopathic and chiropractic examiners, and the basic science boards themselves.

The majority of attorneys general in the basic science states believed that the laws had accomplished their purposes, varied as they seemed to be, and that they had prevented cultists and quacks from flourishing. On the other hand, opinions were divided as to whether or not the laws had helped in the prosecution of illegal practitioners. The majority thought that they could have been prosecuted just as effectively without them.

In the states not having basic science laws the majority of attorneys general did not believe that they were desirable and did not think that law enforcement was handicapped in any respect by their lack. The most succinct reply from an attorney general was, "Dear Doctor, What is a basic science law?" I should like to believe that this showed the unimportance of the laws rather than the ignorance of the respondent.

The replies from the osteopaths of the basic science states expressed no unanimity of opinion as to details of the function of the laws. But the majority did not think they should be repealed. The answers from the osteopaths in the non-basic science states continued the trend—they did not want the laws and saw no advantage in them.

There was a tendency among chiropractors in the basic science states to feel that they were being persecuted. Many of them correctly thought that the laws were deliberately intended to exclude them from licensure and practice. Others, with an air of triumph, stated that basic science laws had definitely improved their educational standards and so they readily accepted the challenge. One chiropractor said that the basic science laws had not achieved their purposes because "many doctors fail, chiropractors pass." An elaboration of this statement would have been interesting.

The chiropractors in the states without basic science laws were unanimous in their condemnation of them.

The majority of the secretaries of the basic science boards believed that they were making worthwhile contributions both to law enforcement and to the elevation of standards. There were only two who thought the laws should be repealed.

The medical profession understandably is concerned over the high failure rate on the basic science examinations. Although it is difficult to learn the number of M.D.'s who fail, as most boards refuse to divulge the identities of the candidates, it is obvious from the statistics published annually by the American Medical Association that the overall rate is high. Furthermore, it is certain that many qualified physicians fail as evidenced by the cries of anguish heard by secretaries of state boards of medical examiners. The overall rate varies from 75 per cent down to seven per cent. The situation is complicated by the fact that certain states have consistently low failure rates and these have broad reciprocity which adds further to the lack of uniformity of standards. Ellis,* with the assistance of the biographical section of the American Medical Association, by a laborious process of elimination, was able to arrive at a reasonably accurate idea of the failure rate of M.D.'s in

* Personal communication.

New Mexico. From 1961 through 1966 the overall failure rate was 64.9 per cent. The failure rate of M.D.'s on their initial attempts was 37 per cent. However, many of these persisted and retook the examination so that their final failure rate was 20 per cent. Although the exact figures are not available, the majority of the candidates who failed were graduates of approved North American medical schools. Lest the reader think that this indicates a breakdown in medical education, I hasten to add that the lack of success of qualified physicians can be partly accounted for by the capriciousness of the policies of the board. For example, I know of one candidate with impeccable qualifications who was temporarily unable to accept a position on the staff of a clinic because he failed the basic science examination in chemistry. By all the rules of common sense he should not have been required to take the examination anyway, as he already had a certificate in another state. But he reckoned without a stupid technicality which stood in the way of reciprocity. The candidate, thinking he would be examined in biochemistry, was confronted by a preponderance of questions in industrial chemistry—good for an engineer but of little importance to a practicing phsyician. Three months later, our candidate, by now an expert in industrial chemistry, repeated the examination which then consisted mainly of biochemistry; he passed. Of course he was not gainfully employed during his enforced absence from practice but during this period he did pass the examinations of the American Board of Pediatrics.

Other reasons for failure are insufficient study because of overconfidence or lack of time. It is difficult for a busy physician 10 or 15 years out of school to go back and study the fine points of chemistry and anatomy.

Until recently, in the many public and private discussions I have held concerning the basic science laws, I have been repeatedly confronted by the supposedly unanswerable argument, "If basic science laws are so bad, why is it that not one has been repealed?" Admittedly this has been difficult to answer. Today, however, I can say that in four states the laws have been repealed. In 1967 the legislature of Florida repealed the basic science law; but this did not become effective until 1969. In January 1968 the New Mexico basic science law was repealed; to the repealer was attached an emergency clause which meant that it would become effective immediately after the governor had signed it. This he did early in February, thus eliminating a useless barrier to licensure of qualified physicians in a state which urgently needs more doctors. Also in January 1968 the legislature of Arizona repealed the law. Alaska repealed its basic science law in 1969. I hope that this is the beginning of a trend and that eventually all basic science laws will be repealed. So far only one other state, Michigan, has attempted such a step and it was defeated on the basis that "high standards must be maintained."

The state medical societies which originally sponsored the basic science laws under the delusion that they were for the public good should reconsider and conduct thorough studies to determine to what extent the laws have succeeded; they should also decide whether it is worthwhile to impose penalties in the form of delay and additional expense upon qualified physicians who are forced to pay a great price to support the mistaken idea that the quacks are being controlled. Already many people have learned that quackery, while it may be discouraged, cannot be controlled by any type of legislation. Furthermore, the charlatan, since the beginning of time, has been sought out by many people, some of whom have become disillusioned by the medical profession. The strongest answer to quackery is the unrestricted movement of qualified physicians about the country permitting them to practice in areas in which they are desperately needed. The basic science laws hinder this; moreover they contribute little or nothing to high standards of medical care. They can only be regarded as anachronistic barriers to the licensure of physicians.

Although I cannot obtain substantiating figures, I am certain that many physicians, particularly those who completed their training from 10 to 15 years previously, refuse to submit to the basic science requirement and so do not settle in states which have these laws. Several of the basic science states have the most acute need for more physicians, yet they permit this barrier to licensure of qualified people to remain. Many physicians have told me that sitting for extra examinations is not worth the time and trouble required.

Whatever useful purpose basic science laws might have served is in the distant past. They should either be repealed or modified so that they cannot continue to exact a penalty from qualified physicians in the form of pointless harassment.

Bibliography

Bierring, W. L. 1930. The Relation of Basic Science Examinations to Medical Licensure. *Fed. Bull.* 16:105–10.

Carter, C. 1941. Basic Science Boards. *Fed. Bull.* 27:79–82.

Clements, L. P. 1943. Basic Science Laws. *Journ. Amer. Med. Coll.* 18:105–12.

Crowe, T. J. 1942. Have Basic Science Medical Laws Advanced Practice of Medicine? *Fed. Bull.* 28:137–41.

Derbyshire, R. C. 1963. Current Attitudes Toward Basic Science Laws. *Fed. Bull.* 50:223–33.

———. 1965. Should There Be Basic Science Boards? *Fed. Bull.* 52:49–61.

DuBois, J. F. 1938. Basic Science Law: Purpose and Effect on Registration and Reciprocity. *Fed. Bull.* 24:171–73.

Federation of State Medical Boards of the United States. 1928. Basic Science Boards. *Fed. Bull.* 14:193–94.

———. 1961. Minutes of Annual Meeting. *Fed. Bull.* 48:146.

Guyer, M. F. 1926. Wisconsin State Board of Examiners in the Basic Sciences. *Fed. Bull.* 12:84–89.

Madison, O. E. 1943. Basic Science Laws, Boards, and Practices in United States. *Fed. Bull.* 29:229–42.

———. 1947. Proposed Uniform Basic Science Laws. *Fed. Bull.* 32:330–44.

Platter, H. M. 1946. Relation of Basic Sciences to Licensure. *Fed. Bull.* 32:164–68.

Taylor, J. G. 1931. Operation of the Basic Science Law in Wisconsin. *Fed. Bull.* 17:140–42.

Woodward, W. C. 1929. The Ineffectiveness of Medical Practice Acts; Basic Science Acts as a Remedy. *Fed. Bull.* 13:267–74.

CHAPTER TEN

THE PROBLEM OF THE
FOREIGN MEDICAL GRADUATE

Fifty years ago, if anyone interested in medical education had encountered the title, "The Problem of the Foreign Medical Graduate," he would have registered puzzlement if not disbelief. "What problem?" he would have asked. For the Flexner report was then only eight years old and the American medical schools were just completing the reforms recommended by its author. American physicians still regarded European medical schools and clinics as superior; any American specialist worthy of the title had at some time in his career been exposed to postgraduate education in Europe.

Furthermore, although the Nobel Prizes in Medicine were conceived in 1901, it was not until 1912 that one was awarded an American—Alexis Carrel—and he had been educated in Europe (Sampey, 1967). During the next 21 years, only two more Americans were so honored, one of whom had been educated in Europe. In 1933 the first graduate of an American university became a Nobel laureate. Although America has rapidly caught up and by now has provided a total of 32 laureates, 10 of them were educated in Europe.

Even today, anyone unfamiliar with the recent history of the European medical schools cannot fully understand why a problem of foreign graduates should exist. Between 1850 and 1913 German medical education was unmatched anywhere in the world. Under the influence of the Germans the same policy of university-type medical education spread to other European countries causing a rapid rise in standards. But the European medical schools could not escape the dislocation of all education caused by World War I, although a few managed to maintain their standards. It remained for Hitler to administer the coup de grâce to the medical schools both by invasion of neighboring countries and the holocaust of World War II. In addition to physical difficulties der Führer imposed his unique ideas for the abbreviated training of ersatz physicians.

Meanwhile, in the United States, medicine along with other phases of life was in the grip of the Great Depression. Medical educators as well as representatives of organized medicine were concerned about the overproduction of physicians, for many of whom there was no apparent room. There were authenticated stories about well-trained physicians who were forced to supplement their meager incomes by selling neckties at Macy's department store. At the same time the German schools were producing poorly trained doctors at an ever increasing rate. Since many could not find work in their own country, they looked to the United States. An additional problem was caused by the graduates of Russian schools whose quality had been questionable even before 1917. The problem was compounded by the poor quality of many of the Central and South American Schools.

In 1930, 167 graduates of foreign medical schools were examined by state boards of medical examiners in the United States with a failure rate of 44.9 per cent. By 1936 the number examined had risen to 644. Concern over the fact that the physician population of the United States was increasing faster than the general population was expressed at the Congress on Medical Education and Licensure by Pinkham in 1938. At the same time he pointed to the difficulty of verification of medical credentials emanating from Germany and Russia. He said, "Frequently products of German medical schools file a large document printed in Latin on thin paper and showing in the lower margin what purports to be the seal of the institution, also printed. Such a document is supposedly a copy of the applicant's original diploma. When questioned, he explains that his original diploma is kept in the archives of the university." He wondered how many alleged medical school products were foisted on the public via a print shop.

Since the beginning of the problem of the foreign medical graduate, New York State has had to cope with the largest number. According to Lochner (1948) from the beginning of the influx in 1926, their failure rate on state board examinations has been high. For example, from June 1945 through February 1947 it was 72 to 78 per cent. Lochner continues, "The attitude of foreign graduates is [characterized by] arrogance and superiority. They resent being required to show their credentials and being required to pass an examination. They try to exert much political pressure." The New York Board of Medical Examiners finally decided that medical education begun in Europe after January 1940 would not be recognized for admission to the licensing examination: possible exceptions were graduates of Cambridge, London and Dublin, medical schools which presumably had standards equal to those of American schools.

By 1935 California had recognized the existence of the foreign graduate problem. Pinkham (1938) pointed out the urgent need for greater uniformity in standards and methods of evaluating the credentials of foreign graduates.

The Federation of State Medical Boards of the United States in 1933 adopted a resolution which would have required that foreign graduates comply with standards of preliminary education established by the Association of American Medical Colleges and the Council on Medical Education and Hospitals of the American Medical Association, with the added requirement that each foreign medical school graduate must hold a license to practice in the country where his school was located. Later the Federation passed a resolution recommending that all graduates of foreign medical schools serve at least one year of internship in an approved United States hospital or complete the senior year of an approved United States medical school. Pinkham found by questionnaire that the latter policy was enforced by only one state board. The California Board was advised by counsel that such a requirement was illegal because the board could not write into the law any requirement that had not been passed by the legislature.

By 1935 seven states and territories—Alaska, Arizona, Georgia, Kentucky, Louisiana, Mississippi and North Carolina—had solved the problem of the foreign graduates by refusing to admit them to their examinations.

The state boards which did admit foreign graduates employed various methods of evaluating credentials. These varied from dependence upon the American Medical Association to correspondence with the rectors of the universities; others relied upon information gathered by the American consuls in the countries concerned. A few reported that they had no method. Systems of examining foreign graduates at this time of necessity varied; unique was the situation in Texas and New Mexico whose boards permitted the candidates to use the assistance of interpreters in taking the examinations.

After 1935 the number of foreign graduates seeking to practice in the United States continued to increase sharply. In addition there was the increasing problem of the American citizens who, for various reasons, were unable to gain admission to North American schools. They were welcomed by many of the foreign schools, many of them of dubious quality. This situation became even more acute after World War II when veterans, under the G.I. Bill of Rights, were permitted to attend foreign schools despite the warnings of the various licensing agencies to the Veterans Administration that graduates of foreign schools would have trouble in obtaining licenses in the United States.

Meanwhile, concern over the problem of the foreign graduate became more widespread. While most medical boards were primarily concerned with the maintenance of standards, others voiced the xenophobia of a certain segment of the medical profession; for example, Vest (1947) made a strong plea that only American citizens be licensed. He argued that at least five years were required for foreign graduates to become familiar with American customs. With questionable accuracy he said that only in rare instances were foreign graduates familiar with the language. In terms prophetic of later attitudes he cried, "It is superfluous to say that American medical practice, medical education, medical ideals, and medical ethics are the best the world has ever known. The influx of alien physicians cannot but lower our professional level."

Many other less eloquent authorities were troubled by the danger that a huge influx of poorly trained foreign graduates would lower American standards. For instance, Furstenberg in 1955 said, "After half a century of unremitting efforts to raise the standards of medical education, licensure, and practice in the United States, we face a threat to further progress if not a substantial loss of qualities already achieved. I refer to graduates of foreign medical schools who are migrating in increasing numbers to this country and who by every measure of our standards have pursued an educational program inferior to those offered in the United States and Canada. . . . Members of our medical faculty [Michigan] are in general agreement that the vast majority of foreign graduates in medicine with whom they have had daily contacts are no match intellectually for the young graduates from our schools at home."

Michigan was one of the first states to require foreign graduates to serve at least a year in an approved United States internship or to take the fourth year of medicine in an approved school. Furstenberg, in relating the 18 years' policy of the University of Michigan School of Medicine in admitting them to the fourth year class, said, "Our experience with the majority of them was discouraging and sometimes futile."

Schnoor (1955), also from Michigan, said, "Apparent doctor-shortage propaganda has produced sympathetic public appeal for more doctors without due consideration of presently attained American standards as foreign doctors are encouraged to enter the United States. Michigan, because of its experience with the early group of foreign graduates, the displaced persons, pioneered in definite efforts both to help the foreign graduates and to prevent the poorly trained ones from lowering American standards." The Board of Medical Examiners, in cooperation with the medical schools of the University of Michigan and Wayne State University, developed a screening board composed of 12 medical educators, half from each school. The foreign graduate applying for licensure who met

the usual requirements but with doubtful educational background was referred to the screening board on a voluntary basis
for an oral comprehensive examination. During the first three
years of its existence 186 examinations were given, including
25 re-examinations. At first the screening process was applied
only to the displaced physicians. But soon the following
additional classes of foreign graduates had to be considered:
1. The permanent émigré. 2. The émigré on a temporary visa
for postgraduate education. 3. The American citizen who had
received his medical education in a substandard medical
school. 4. A small group of doctors licensed in other states
who wished to enter Michigan by endorsement, but had
graduated from unapproved foreign medical schools. Dr.
Schnoor, then the president of the Michigan Board of Medical
Examiners, expressed satisfaction with the screening tests and
found good correlation between the candidates' grades on
these and on the examinations of the Board of Medical
Examiners.

At about the same time the authorities in New York
State developed a one year intensive course for foreign graduates at New York University. Boggs (1955), in describing this,
admitted the difficulty of giving the equivalent of four years of
training in one year. He also pointed to their mistake with the
first class with no effort at selection. The succeeding classes
were carefully screened for aptitude, educational background,
and knowledge of English. "In summary," said Boggs, "we
found our task arduous but extremely rewarding. . . . It is our
considered opinion that the great majority of the immigrant
physicians, with supplemental medical education, can meet
the high standards that we demand for practice in this country."

During this period the American Medical Association had
not been idle and had attempted partially to meet the problem
of the foreign graduate. In 1950 the AMA's Council on
Medical Education published a list of foreign medical schools
whose graduates were recommended for consideration on a
comparable basis with that of graduates of approved American
schools. This list was welcomed as a guide by boards of
medical examiners which had no means of evaluating foreign

schools. Many foreign graduates were admitted to examinations on the strength of having been graduated from "approved foreign schools." According to Wiggins (1955), 68 per cent of these candidates were successful in passing the state board examinations, while only 46 per cent of graduates of unlisted schools passed. But, to the dismay of many licensing boards, the list was withdrawn after ten years.

The reasons for the withdrawal of the list were ably summarized by Smiley (1955) who wrote, "First it was felt that any system of quasi accrediting based upon the happenstance of an American medical educator's visit to a foreign school was altogether too fortuitous to be either fair or defensible; second, it was felt that if a school were to be fairly evaluated, it would have to be visited by a team of medical educators and formally surveyed, just as our American schools are surveyed; third, it was felt that even if the funds were available to do it, it would still be unwise and fraught with unsurmountable difficulties for medical educators from this country to evaluate medical education programs of other countries whose cultural, economic, and educational backgrounds were so different from ours."

By 1955 the problem of proper evaluation of the foreign graduate had become a national concern. The reasons for this were summarized by Smiley who pointed out that the situation was different from the days when American students flocked to European centers for advanced training. The American students did not serve on house staffs of hospitals nor did they assume responsibility for treatment of patients without first passing the local licensing examinations. But in the United States, in 1955, physicians trained in some 83 countries were permitted to practice in American hospitals with neither a license nor any real evaluation of their previous medical training. Smiley stressed the completely theoretical training given by many foreign schools which register several hundred students in each class. He concluded that such lack of evaluation constituted a real threat to the safety and well being of hospital patients cared for by these foreign graduates. He called for an effective examination system.

At about the same time the Cooperating Council for the Evaluation of Foreign Medical Schools was formed. Sponsors were the American Medical Association's Council on Medical Education, the Association of American Medical Colleges, the Federation of State Medical Boards of the United States, and the American Hospital Association. This was the precursor of the Educational Council for Foreign Medical Graduates which was formed in 1956, and began to function on October 1, 1957. Members of its board include representatives of the founding organizations and, in addition, two members from the public at large. "Its stated purpose is to provide information to foreign medical graduates, to verify credentials, and to evaluate the educational qualifications of foreign trained physicians who desire to advance their education in the United States, and to arrange examinations to determine the readiness of such individuals to benefit from education in U.S. hospitals" (AMA, 1967).

The Council's examinations consist essentially of three parts: 1. Examination of the educational background of foreign graduates to determine that they have had at least 18 years of formal education including adequate time spent in medical school. 2. A test of the candidates' ability to understand English. 3. A test of the candidates' knowledge of medicine. Until 1966 the Educational Council annually made the statement that possession of its certificate was evidence that a candidate's school was equal to American schools. However, this was obviously inaccurate and caused much misunderstanding and ill feeling both on the part of foreign graduates and boards of medical examiners. Therefore, the statement was revised to read as follows: "That agencies in the United States concerned with medical qualifications of graduates of foreign medical schools consider certification by the Educational Council for Foreign Medical Graduates as evidence that the recipients of such certification have medical knowledge at least comparable with the minimum expected of graduates of approved medical schools in the United States and Canada." (AMA, 1967).

Although primarily founded to help teaching hospitals select qualified foreign graduates as members of their house staffs, the Educational Council for Foreign Medical Graduates is now performing a service for the boards of medical examiners as well. The boards themselves find it impossible to classify foreign medical schools. When the American Medical Association withdrew its list of approved foreign schools some other method of screening of foreign graduates became necessary. Consequently many of the boards began to use the certificate of the Educational Council for this purpose. While four boards, those of Connecticut, Kentucky, Maine, and Minnesota, maintain their own lists of approved foreign schools, the majority of the remaining states, 43 in number, require that candidates for board examinations possess certificates of the Council.

The reasons that the boards of medical examiners view the certificate of the Educational Council as evidence of screening only are obvious. Although the medical examinations are compiled from questions of the National Board of Medical Examiners, they are not the same examinations that are given to graduates of American schools applying for standard certification. Even so only 40 per cent of foreign graduates pass on the first try: the scores of those who do pass are mainly just above the passing level with only a few higher.

The performance of foreign graduates on state board examinations is equally discouraging, the failure rate being 38.2 per cent compared with 4.2 per cent for United States graduates and 11.7 per cent for Canadians (AMA, 1967). The latter are not classified as foreign graduates as their schools are accredited by the same agencies that inspect United States schools.

Despite the academic difficulties and dubious quality of many foreign graduates, we must face the fact that for several years they have been occupying an increasingly important place in the practice of medicine in the United States. Today there is a definite shortage of physicians in this country and foreign graduates are helping to alleviate it. Since 1950, 18,400 foreign graduates representing additions to the medical profession have been licensed. Since 1957 they have been licensed at the rate of from 1,000 to 1,500 a year. This is roughly equivalent to the output of 12 medical schools and represents 18 per cent of the annual addition to the medical profession. According to West (1965) if the true cost of building and operating that many schools is calculated, "The dollar value per year of this 'foreign aid' to the United States approximately equals the total cost of all of our medical aid, private and public, to foreign nations."

Many authorities believe that the main purpose of bringing foreign graduates to the United States is to give them needed postgraduate education in order that they can improve medical standards when they return to their home countries. But large numbers choose to remain in the United States to practice. Hunt (1966) refers to this as "The Brain Drain in Medicine." He voices the opinion of many others that a sufficient number of American doctors must be educated to meet the needs of the American people. India, in 1967, became so concerned about the loss of her physicians to the United States that the authorities refused to permit the Educational Council for Foreign Medical Graduates to conduct examinations in the country.

What about the foreign graduate who has fulfilled all of the strict requirements, passed his state board examination and has finally become fully licensed in a state? Even though he has attained full citizenship, can he regard himself as a true member of the American medical profession? Unfortunately, the answer is no, particularly if he chooses to stray from the state in which he is licensed and seeks to become qualified in another. Although most of these states will license by endorsement American graduates, the rules are far different where the foreign graduate is concerned. He will find a bewildering array of laws, rules, and regulations which he will be certain were designed to plague him personally. But, lest he become paranoid, let me point out that these apply to all foreign graduates. He will find that in three states, Arkansas, Louisiana, and Nevada, he will not be accepted under any circumstances. Neither Lord Lister nor Billroth could have practiced in these states, not to mention such modern European giants of the profession as Sir Reginald Watson-Jones, Sir Heneage Ogilvie and Professor Clarence Craaford.

Questionnaire Sent to States Which Refuse to License Foreign Medical Graduates by Endorsement

1. Is your refusal to license foreign graduates by endorsement due to law or board policy? (Law–14; Board policy–11.)

2. Why do you refuse to license foreign graduates by endorsement? (Because law does not permit–8; No direct answers–4; Board has no confidence in examinations of other boards–4; Board wishes to know candidates' plans for practicing in state–2; Legislative intent unknown–1; Must have true reciprocity–1; Impossible to classify answers–5.)

3. If a foreign graduate could meet your other requirements and had passed the Federation Licensing Examination with standard scores, would you consider him for licensure by endorsement? (Yes–5; No–19; Do not know–1.)

4. If a world-famous medical scientist or professor, a foreign graduate, applied for licensure by endorsement would you make an exception for him? (Yes–3; No–22.)

In the jurisdictions* in which our qualified foreign graduate might be accepted, he will find that there are many variations in citizenship requirements; in 25 he must be a full citizen, in 20 he must have filed a declaration of intention, while in 10 there are not citizenship requirements at all. In addition, in 20 states he must pass a basic science examination before he can be even considered for licensure examination. And if he wishes to obtain a license by endorsement he must make careful inquiries, since in only 13 states can he do this; in the remaining 38 he must take another examination. Although most medical practice acts state that endorsement can be granted only if standards are equal, frequently lip service only is paid to this requirement where graduates of American schools are concerned. Regarding foreign graduates, however, George Orwell's parallel from *The Animal Farm* is apt, "All animals are equal but some animals are more equal than others."

* Under this term are included the Canal Zone, Guam, Virgin Islands, and Puerto Rico in addition to the states and the District of Columbia.

By careful inquiry the foreign graduate might learn of other stumbling blocks. These range from one which requires five years of residency in an approved United States hospital to lengthy statements concerning the physical equipment and curriculum of his school. He might be consoled by the fact that in one state (South Dakota) he would not starve while waiting his five years to obtain the required full citizenship; he would have to work in the state mental hospital. Particularly interesting is the requirement of two states, Alabama and Utah, that he must have a certificate from the National Board of Medical Examiners; in view of the fact that the National Board stopped examining foreign graduates in 1952, for all practical purposes these states must be added to the list of the three refusing to license foreign graduates.

The restrictions on the mobility of fully licensed foreign graduates is understandably a source of bewilderment and frustration to them. One of the more vocal, a foreign-born, foreign-educated, naturalized citizen, a member of the American Medical Association, a board certified specialist, licensed in a state by examination, complains because other states will not endorse his license even though they will accept those of Canadian and American graduates from his state (Derbyshire,

Table 8. Additional Requirements for Licensure of Foreign Medical Graduates

ECFMG Certificate	44 jurisdictions
Full Citizenship	27 jurisdictions
Declaration of Intention	20 jurisdictions
No citizenship requirements	8 jurisdictions
Basic Science Certificate	22 jurisdictions

Educational Requirements

One year approved internship	4 jurisdictions
Two year internship or residency	10 jurisdictions
Three year residency	4 jurisdictions
Five year residency	1 jurisdiction
Residency training as specified by board	1 jurisdiction
At least one year of training must be in state	3 jurisdictions
Considered on individual basis	7 jurisdictions
Certificate of National Board of Medical Examiners	3 jurisdictions

1966). He laments the fact that the foreign graduate remains eternally stigmatized in the name of states' rights and despite membership in any number of professional societies he remains a second class citizen. The foreign graduate, although he passes the same examination and obtains the same certificate as do graduates of North American schools, is treated entirely differently when he seeks endorsement in another state. One such physician said, "The students and interns I teach are given more consideration by the boards than I am."

By what logic do so many state boards consign the foreign graduate to the eternal status of second class citizen? One explanation is the lack of confidence of state boards in the quality of the examinations of other states. In addition they do not entirely trust the screening system of the Educational Council. The ability to pass any number of examinations cannot substitute for sound medical education in a first class medical school. Furthermore, there is wide variation in the standards and methods of many state boards. For example, there are at least nine states which practically never fail a candidate; others use the National Board questions but set a lower passing level, while the questions of some states are archaic and obviously written by people not familiar with the specialties. Also many state boards, from their observation of the performance of some foreign graduates both on examinations and in practice, believe that neither screening nor licensure in another state provides assurance of quality.

One possible answer to the problem of inadequate screening is to raise the standards of the Educational Council for Foreign Medical Graduates so that the certificate might serve as an authoritative statement of equality of training to that of American graduates. Many state boards would welcome such a change. But, despite the fact that the Federation of State Medical Boards is one of the sponsoring organizations, the Council still feels primarily obligated to the hospitals. If the standards of the Council were raised the failure rate would soar far above its present 60 per cent, thus depriving many hospitals of much-needed help. A recent attempt to raise standards was blocked for this reason.

The questionable ability of many foreign graduates who have passed the examinations of the Educational Council gives pause to boards of medical examiners. The language difficulty alone is sufficient to make them wonder just what kind of examination the foreign graduates have passed. A story, possibly apocryphal, which recently made the rounds concerns the foreign graduate who failed in his English examination. The hospital which intended to employ him interceded with the defense that he was to be an orthopedics resident and so did not need to know any English!

Although the recurrent evidence of double standards upsets both educators and licensing boards, the Educational Council for Foreign Medical Graduates does fulfill a certain function, for it spares the licensing boards the necessity of examining large numbers of obviously hopeless candidates.

Recently still another agency became concerned over the problem of the foreign medical graduate. The National Advisory Commission on Health Manpower, in its report to the President (1967) stated that foreign medical graduates with less education and lower test ratings than those required of United States graduates are allowed to assume responsibilities for the care of patients. It points to the fact that the examination of the Educational Council for Foreign Medical Graduates is easier than that of the National Board. The scores of foreign graduates on state board examinations are poor; even after training in this country, examinations which were passed by 96 per cent of graduates of United States schools were passed by only 40 per cent of foreign graduates. The report continues, "This figure has added importance because those who do not pass frequently remain in the United States, working in jobs for which the requirements for licensure are waived (e.g., many states do not require that physicians in state hospitals be licensed)."

The Health Manpower Commission recommends that foreign-trained physicians who will have responsibility for patient care be required to pass tests equivalent to those for graduates of U.S. schools; for this it suggests use of the examinations of the National Board of Medical Examiners. It also advocates that foreign graduates participate in an orientation and educational program in which their competence could be assessed and necessary remedial instruction provided.

American citizens who are graduates of foreign medical schools present their own problems. Accurate data concerning the number of Americans who go to foreign countries for their medical education are difficult to obtain. However, the Institute of International Education estimated that in 1963–64 approximately 1,643 were enrolled in foreign schools. Greeley (1966) estimated that about 500 to 550 Americans start in medical schools in foreign countries each year, while 300 graduate and take the E. C. F. M. G. examinations.

Americans attend foreign medical schools for a variety of reasons. A few do not apply to American schools at all and apparently prefer to study abroad. But the majority are unable to obtain admission to American schools as evidenced by the fact that many of them have been rejected by as many as seven to ten. This is because of their poor academic records in college and their low scores on the Medical College Admissions Tests. Still others, because of financial difficulties or for other reasons, decide only late in life to study medicine. Many of these apparently are determined individuals and I have known several of them who, at the age of 40 or more years, applied to several American medical schools only to be turned down mainly on the basis of age. But their determination was so great that they grasped at any foreign school regardless of quality, thinking that their problems would be solved merely by the acquisition of any M.D. degree. But after graduation many of them are unable to pass the examinations of the E. C. F. M. G., much less those of the boards of medical examiners.

Greeley, in his study of American foreign medical graduates, substantiated the above impressions. He found that the 72 per cent of American foreign graduates who had been rejected by American schools had significantly lower test scores on the Medical College Aptitude Tests than those students who were accepted by American schools. He further learned that after graduation from foreign schools, 57 per cent passed the E. C. F. M. G. examinations on the first try, while 70 per cent eventually passed it after one or more additional attempts. This leaves a total of 30 per cent or some 90 students each year who can never obtain licenses to practice in the United States. Unable or unwilling to practice in foreign countries, they find themselves medical men without countries who have wasted precious years of their lives because of their ill-advised efforts to become doctors.

On the other hand, there is one bright spot in the dreary picture of the American foreign graduate. At present a few selected students who have made good academic records in foreign schools are being accepted as transfer students in the third year classes of some American schools. This enables them to obtain acceptable American M.D. degrees. Recently the National Board of Medical Examiners agreed to help in the identification of the more gifted students by allowing them to take Part I of its examination. But by no means has the Board opened its examinations to all who would take them and has agreed only to examine those who have been recommended by the Association of American Medical Colleges.

It is far easier to describe the problem of the foreign graduate than to solve it. But two aspects are particularly clear; first, poorly trained physicians must not be allowed to lower the standards of medical care in the United States. This could be partially prevented by the elimination of the double standard and by requiring all foreign graduates to pass the same standardized tests of high quality required of United States graduates. Second, a natural sequel would be the elimination of discrimination against properly licensed and qualified foreign graduates which restricts their mobility and limits their opportunities. This can be done only if the state boards of medical examiners establish uniformly high standards thereby restoring their confidence in the examinations of other states.

Bibliography

American Medical Association. 1967. State Board Number. *J.A.M.A.* 200:1079.

Boggs, R. 1955. Supplementary Medical Education for Immigrant Physicians. *Fed. Bull.* 41:137–42.

Derbyshire, R. C. 1966. The Problem of Multiple Standards. *Fed. Bull.* 53:108–17.

Federation of State Medical Boards of the United States. 1966. Minutes of the Annual Business Meeting. *Fed. Bull.* 53:257–58.

Furstenberg, A. C. 1955. The Evaluation of Foreign Medical Graduates for Licensure. *Fed. Bull.* 41:123–42.

Greeley, D. McL. 1966. American Foreign Medical Graduates. *J. Med. Educ.* 41:641–50.

Hunt, G. H. 1966. The Brain Drain in Medicine. *Fed. Bull.* 53:98.

Institute of International Education. 1965. *Open Doors Report on International Exchange.* New York. Quoted by Greeley.

Lochner, J. L. 1948. Licensure Evaluation of European Medical Graduates. *J.A.M.A.* 137:16–17.

Orwell, G. 1947. *Animal Farm.* New York: Harcourt, Brace and Company.

Pinkham, C. B. 1938. Foreign Medical Students. *Fed. Bull.* 24:132–52.

Report of the National Advisory Commission on Health Manpower. 1967. Washington: U. S. Government Printing Office.

Sampey, J. R. 1967. Academic Backgrounds of Nobel Laureates in Medicine and Physiology. *J. Med. Educ.* 42:1126.

Schnoor, E. W. 1955. Today Is Not Yesterday: The Problem of the Foreign Medical Graduate. *Fed. Bull.* 41:110–22.

Smiley, D. F. 1955. *J. Med. Educ.* 30:588.

Vest, W. E. 1947. Citizenship as Related to Licensure. *Fed. Bull.* 28:100–107.

West, K. M. 1965. Foreign Interns and Residents in the United States. *J. Med. Educ.* 40:1127.

Wiggins, W. S. 1955. Proposed Program for the Evaluation of Graduates of Foreign Medical Schools. *Fed. Bull.* 41:150–67.

CHAPTER ELEVEN

THE NEED FOR
A NEW APPROACH

In 1888 the *Journal of the American Medical Association* published a letter from Dr. William Osler which referred to a report of the Medical Examining Board of Virginia. Dr. Osler said, "It is not the function of the University to grant the license to practice but it is the function of the State to be exercised by the profession organizing and appointing suitable examiners." This was in the pre-Flexner days and he believed that boards of medical examiners could establish minimal requirements for medical practice for the protection of the public.

But 14 years later Osler (*see* Osler, 1944), speaking in Canada about the barriers erected by state and provincial licensing boards said, ". . . it is provincialism run riot. That this pestiferous condition should exist throughout the various provinces of this Dominion and in many states of the Union illustrates what I have said of the tyranny of democracy and how great enslavers of liberty its chief proclaimers may be."

What happened between 1888 and 1902 to have caused such an outburst from a former champion of state boards of medical examiners? The boards had been partially successful in protecting the public against the depredations of ill-trained graduates of inferior schools. But somehow they added to their original function by building walls around their states which hampered the free movement of qualified physicians. In 1968 would Osler still refer to "this pestiferous condition"? I believe he would, for many barriers to interstate endorsement of medical licenses still exist, be they based on socio-economic or academic considerations or mere caprice.

For many years the Federation of State Medical Boards of the United States has been mainly concerned with the establishment of universal reciprocity or endorsement among the states.* In fact, certain members have become so shrill in voicing their demands that they have lost sight of the fact that most state laws carefully spell out the requirement that endorsement can be offered only to those states which have standards equal to their own. In other words, these strident advocates of endorsement at any price believe that relationships should be based on nothing firmer than mutual admiration and gentlemen's agreements. Consequently, the few states which interpreted their statutes literally found themselves unable to endorse the licenses of many states whose standards are far from equal.

New York is a notable example of the states which insist upon equal requirements and thereby has not endeared itself to the advocates of universal endorsement. However, this state has elevated standards by causing the boards of some other states to take a hard look at the quality of their examinations. For example, among the examination questions of one state which were considered inadequate by New York were, "State the source of ichthyol and its uses in medicine" and, "Give the common name, the source, and the principal therapeutic uses of oleum theobroma." These questions, when asked today in the last half of the twentieth century, no doubt struck terror into the hearts of recent medical graduates. I must add that this state was finally approved by New York, but only after attrition had eliminated the senior citizen who originated such questions.

It is remarkable that any of the boards have been able to endorse the certificates of others. There are vast differences in the subjects included in the examinations; there is lack of uniformity concerning the levels of passing grades, and there is a patchwork of grandfather clauses and bonuses for years of practice. While endorsement is fairly easy for graduates of approved North American medical schools, mutual distrust

* The term "endorsement" is preferable to reciprocity and is now more commonly used as the latter implies contracts relating to mutual interests.

among boards is manifested by their treatment of graduates of foreign medical schools. Although they pass the same state board examinations required of American graduates, they are by no means treated as equals where endorsement is concerned. Aside from the three states which refuse to license foreign graduates under any circumstances, there are 24 which decline to accept them by endorsement, thus relegating them to the permanent status of second class medical citizens.

Another example of the lack of uniformity of standards has been the variable failure rate among the various state boards. In 1961 Hubbard stated that in 1958 nearly half of the state boards reported no failures in the examinations of 2,000 physicians, and he pointed to the difficulty of having confidence in the examinations of a state board with a reputation for giving easy examinations. In 1965 I pursued this question further and studied the failure rates in state board examinations for the preceding ten years. I found that three state boards had not failed a single candidate during this period; two states did not fail anyone in nine out of ten years; four reported no failures in eight out of ten years. Furthermore, the six states in the last two categories had low rates in the years in which they did report failures, usually less than two per cent. The nine states with the lowest failure rates for ten years examined a total of 10,455 candidates, failing only 14, a rate of less than .014 per cent. These candidates were not all native sons; many graduates of foreign medical schools were also examined.*

Two years later I brought the study up to date. The number of lenient boards had dropped from nine to three but there were still two which reported no failures for 12 consecutive years. During this period they examined a total of 2,219 candidates (Derbyshire, 1966).

* The lenient states were Oklahoma, Idaho, Tennessee, Kentucky, Wyoming, Michigan, Minnesota, Alabama and South Carolina. When questioned recently by Richard B. Lyons of the *New York Times*, secretaries of some of these boards gave such answers as "applicants for licensure are screened well in advance of the test" and "13 applicants had failed since 1964 but were not listed as failures. They were given a second chance to pass the test and most did."

According to Hoffman (1963), the examination might represent only a formality to the candidate who is applying in the same state in which he attended medical school. In one year 26 state boards did not fail a single local graduate and many boards pass all of them year after year. She called this "native son treatment."

At the opposite extreme are certain states with consistently high failure rates. I arbitrarily selected five states with the highest failure rates during the past five years. Only those examining significant numbers of candidates were studied. I found that during the past five years some states had consistently failed over 40 per cent of the candidates every year. Four states had been on the high failure list every year, while one state was on it for three years. Significant is the fact that the failures in these states were not confined to the foreign graduates but included graduates of North American schools and some went so far as to fail an appreciable number of "native sons." It is amazing that there can be any legal interstate endorsement of licenses with such a wide variation in standards.

To account for the lack of uniformity of standards among the state boards one must examine the composition of the boards themselves. Universally made up of political appointees of either the party or medical variety, they are seldom selected primarily as experts in the various subjects of the examinations. In fact this criterion is often defeated by the statutes of some states which specify that board members cannot belong to the faculties of medical schools. In the few laws which list the qualifications of examiners moral and ethical standards are stressed without mention of academic attainments. No wonder there is lack of uniformity of quality of examinations when a radiologist must examine in gynecology or a general practitioner whose sole claim to academic distinction may be the serving of a one year internship 15 years ago, is asked to examine in physiology or pathology! Moreover, the majority of these examiners have had no training in the technique of examining and no concept as to the validity of their questions.

Another difficulty of board members as examiners is the fact that their important disciplinary and administrative functions tend to overshadow their duty to give high quality examinations.

During much of the 56 years of its existence the Federation of State Medical Boards of the United States has been primarily concerned with legal and administrative matters almost to the exclusion of quality of examinations. Later the problem of the graduates of foreign medical schools had to be faced. But, in the background, there was a widespread feeling of uneasiness due to increasing awareness of the need for careful study of the quality of licensing examinations, and consideration of their part in the educational system. In 1956 these doubts were formulated in a recommendation that a permanent committee be appointed "to develop and activate examination institutes in the major branches of medicine covered in the licensure examinations, for the purpose of creating uniformity in content and quality in these examinations."

In 1956 the original Examination Institute Committee outlined its objectives as follows (*see* Federation of State Medical Boards of the United States, 1961): (1) Uniformity in licensing examinations. (2) Establishment of equivalent levels in the examinations. (3) Improvement in the quality of examinations. (4) Creation of a rational basis for interstate endorsement. (5) Placement of licensure in a definite relation to modern medical education. (6) Assisting state boards in managing the foreign graduate problem.

Undeniably the aims of the original committee were lofty and if accomplished would have improved the quality of state board examinations. Especially significant was the fourth objective, the creation of a rational basis for interstate endorsement. From the first the Committee realized that uniformly high quality of examinations was the most important basis for endorsement.

Also noteworthy was the fifth objective, the placement of the licensure examination in a definite relation to modern education. The Institute Committee assigned the state board examination, in the educational plan, to a place following the internship or residency, a time when it can be safely assumed that the candidate possesses much factual knowledge, the only question being his ability to apply it. Thus the concept of "fitness testing" was conceived and it was agreed that the primary objective of the licensure examination is to determine whether or not the candidate is capable of dealing intelligently with the everyday problems of medical practice.

The first Examination Institute was held in 1957 and since then such institutes have been an annual event. For the first three years major attention was focused on the application of the general concept of fitness testing to the various subjects of the state board examinations including the basic sciences. Broad questions were propounded and many of these of necessity concerned the content of the examinations and the subjects being taught in the medical schools today. While it is difficult to assess the results of the early institutes, the quality of examinations of a few states, at least, was improved to the extent that they could be accepted by New York which continued to require equal standards as a basis for endorsement. On the other hand, a subsequent look at the questions of many other state boards revealed that there was no change in the nature of their questions or improvement in their quality.

To solve the problem of the board member who must examine in a subject outside his field, an experimental pool of questions was developed. Although this gained some acceptance among the boards, it was shelved in 1965 in favor of another plan which, although slow in its development, has at last reached full fruition.

For several years the Examination Institute Committee of the Federation of State Medical Boards has believed that the best method of attaining its objectives was to devise standard examinations of high quality in all of the subjects which could be offered to the individual states. The members of the committee realized that these examinations would have to be pretested for validity, and should be consistent with the concept of fitness testing. If such examinations could be offered and widely accepted by the state boards, interstate endorsement could at last be placed upon a sound basis. Furthermore, every board would know the type of examination each candidate for endorsement had passed. Obviously the establishment of uniform standards could help solve the problems of endorsement of the graduates of foreign medical schools.

The long-standing argument about objective versus essay examinations, while not yet finally laid to rest, has been at least temporarily halted. The extensive studies of the National Board of Medical Examiners proved to the satisfaction of most that their objective methods of testing are reliable and convinced the Institute Committee of their worth.

But before the Federation could offer an acceptable service it had to overcome several obstacles. Although an appraisal of the membership revealed an ample number of talented and discriminating specialists representing several fields, there were few who were familiar with the modern techniques of testing. Also the vagaries of politics preclude assurance of continuity of membership in the Federation. Moreover, to carry out any such plan, financial resources far beyond those of the Federation would have been required. Therefore the Institute Committee called upon the National Board of Medical Examiners for consultation. Although many candidates are licensed on the basis of their National Board certificates, there are still nine states which either refuse to accept the National Board or do so with reservations. Furthermore, the National Board does not examine graduates of foreign medical schools.

After several conferences, the National Board kindly consented to make available to the Federation its vast store of validated, pretested questions with the understanding that the members of the Federation would be allowed to select those best suited to their purpose of fitness testing. A contract was signed whereby the Federation was to be responsible for the administration of the examinations by the individual states, the scoring to be carried out by the National Board. These are truly state board examinations and the booklets are imprinted with the name of the individual state. The National Board sends the scores to the Federation which makes a record of them before sending them to the states. The National Board charges the Federation $57.50 for each examination: the

Federation adds a charge of $7.50 for administrative expenses, making a total of $65.00 for the examination of each candidate.

In October 1967 the Federation test committees met and selected the items for the first Federation examination to be given in June 1968. The members excluded the least difficult questions, as well as the more complicated questions which mainly demanded the recall of knowledge. The examination is given in three parts, each requiring one day. The first day is concerned with the six traditional basic science subjects, 90 items having been selected from each group. The second day 90 test items in the six areas of clinical medicine are presented. The examinations of the first and second days are given in interdisciplinary form; that is, there is no labeling of specific subjects so that the candidates are given "scrambled" examinations. But to comply with state laws, the conventional subjects are extracted and the grades reported to the state boards.

The third day is devoted to testing for clinical competence. For this, items from Part III of the National Board examinations are used. This truly rounds out the concept of fitness testing and gives the state boards an impression as to the ability of the candidates to deal with clinical problems in medical practice. The material is presented by means of pictures of patients or specimens, reproductions of roentgenograms and electrocardiograms, motion pictures of selected patients to test the powers of observation of the candidates and their ability to draw proper conclusions from the material. Also included is that part of the National Board examinations known as programmed testing, designed to assess the judgment of the candidate in sequential management of patients.

Already many questions have been raised concerning the Federation licensing examination, particularly by graduates of foreign medical schools. Some examples and the answers follow: 1. Will the passage of this examination entitle the candidate to a National Board certificate? (It will not.) 2. Will the candidate who passes it be eligible for licensure by endorsement in all of the states? (No; this is an individual state board examination and, until state laws and regulations are changed, the rules for endorsement will remain as they are. The Federation hopes that, since there are to be uniform examinations, universal acceptance of the examinations will eventually bring about broad endorsement policies by all of the states.) 3. Will the passing level be the same in every state? (It will not, as each state reserves the right to set its own passing grades. However, according to Heywood (1968), the true scores will be reported to the Federation and these will be available to any state board requiring them.)

The Federation licensing examination will not duplicate the present services of the National Board. As Heywood (1967) said, "These are entirely new examinations constructed to conform to the Federation's concept of fitness testing." They should be particularly valuable to those states which do not accept the National Board certificate. Moreover, for the first time graduates of foreign medical schools may be evaluated on the basis of standardized examinations of high quality. This should eliminate the prevailing distrust among the state boards. Granted the passing of any number of examinations will not take the place of sound medical training, the majority of foreign graduates take additional training in the United States before applying for licensure. Therefore the Federation licensing examination can provide a means of evaluating their postgraduate training as well as their fundamental ability.

According to Hubbard (1968), more and more state boards are asking the National Board to provide them with questions for use in their own examinations. During 1967 a total of 16 states used such questions in examining 4,584 individuals. But so far these states have used only the questions of Parts I and II. Hubbard said that the staff of the National Board had asked whether the type of test material that was being furnished to these states is "the best that could be provided to meet the oft-declared objective of the Federation to test for fitness for the practice of medicine." In discussing Part III of the National Board examination, he pointed out that it is designed for those who have had experience in the care of patients. He continued, "The methods and content of these objective measurements of clinical competence are very clearly applicable to the objective of state licensing boards in testing for fitness to practice general medicine. Yet . . . no state board is using these procedures for its licensing examination." Hence it is important that a full day of testing of clinical competence be included in the Federation licensing examination.

The Federation Licensing Examinations were first given in 1968; in June and December of that year they were administered to a total of 889 candidates in seven states. In addition, 1969, nine other states—New York, California, Utah, Indiana, Oregon, Montana, Connecticut, and Colorado—are using or planning to use these examinations. Other states are interested but for the moment are unable to use the Federation's examinations. Statutory limitations have proven the most common obstacles to universal use of the examinations. For example, some state laws specify the cost of their examinations which is below that of the Federation; other laws state that essay examinations must be given and some even prescribe the number of questions which must be asked. Although in most cases only minor changes in the statutes would be required, legislatures may be slow in adopting them. Therefore, many years may pass before there can be universal acceptance of the examinations. But this remains the ultimate goal. It is the only conceivable solution to the problem of uniform standards unless all of the states should decide to accept the certificate of the National Board and the Board would consent to examine foreign graduates, both remote possibilities at present.

The present system of state licensure is under attack by many people. Some think that state board examinations should be abolished and the diploma granted by an accredited medical school should entitle a physician to practice. Others favor federal licensure of physicians, with relegation of the state boards to the handling of moral qualifications of applicants and disciplinary matters. The National Advisory Commission on Health Manpower, in its recent report (1967) to President Johnson, recommended that medical licensure be based on minimum requirements throughout the country. It points to a need for research to develop model provisions for licensure problems such as interstate endorsement of licenses. I can find little need for research in this field. The answer to the problem of interstate endorsement has been found; it can only be based upon uniformly high standards.

Milford Rouse, President of the American Medical Association, at a recent annual meeting of the Federation, questioned the necessity of demanding written examinations as a requirement for medical licensure. He also wondered why all of the state boards could not accept the results of the National Board examination as the basis for granting a state license (Rouse, 1968).

Although licensure examinations may have outlived their period of usefulness, they will not be abandoned in the foreseeable future for three reasons; first is the continuing influence of the doctrine of states' rights. Second, the problem of the foreign graduate is still a real one. Third, the establishment of national licensure would require an amendment to the Constitution of the United States. Traditionally licensing has been a function of the state because of the Tenth Amendment which provides that powers not delegated to the United States are reserved to the states or the people. Therefore, the state boards, with the help of their Federation and the National Board, must accept their duty to establish uniform standards of high quality for licensure and interstate endorsement. The mechanism is at hand; the only question is, will it be properly used?

Bibliography

AMA. 1888. Quoted by Bierring, W. L. *Fed. Bull.* 31:162–63.

Derbyshire, R. C. 1965. How to Obtain a License—in One Easy Lesson. *Fed. Bull.* 52:124–27.

———. 1966. An End to Leniency? Editorial, *Fed. Bull.* 52:202–3.

Federation of State Medical Boards of the United States. 1961. *Report on Examination Institutes: 1957–1958–1959.*

Heywood, L. T. 1967. The New Direction. *Fed. Bull.* 54:93.

———. 1968. The Federation Examination. *Fed. Bull.* 55:11–14.

Hoffman, L. 1963. What You Have to Go Through to Get a License! *Riss.* 6:52–62.

Hubbard, J. P. 1961. The Role of Examining Boards in Medical Education and in Qualification for Clinical Practice. *J. Med. Educ.* 36:94–102.

———. 1968. Uniformity of Qualification for Medical Practice and States' Rights. *Fed. Bull.* 55:2–10.

Osler, W. 1944. *Aequanimitas*. Philadelphia: Blakiston Co., p. 276.

Report of the National Advisory Commission on Health Manpower. 1967. Washington: U. S. Government Printing Office.

Rouse, M. O. 1968. Walter L. Bierring Lecture. *Fed. Bull.* 55:73.

CHAPTER TWELVE

CONCLUSIONS

Anyone who discusses medical licensure in America today feels impelled to present the subject against the historical background of licensing in European countries and Great Britain. But licensing in the United States has taken an entirely different turn from the system in England where the acquisition of a medical degree is tantamount to a license to practice medicine. The system in the United States is also entirely different from that in Canada where the one examination of the Medical Council is recognized voluntarily by all of the provinces except Quebec. Medical licensure in the United States is unique in that the laws and regulations have been separately written by some 55 different jurisdictions.

An important historical point is that in the early years of this country, before medical education became a function of the universities, preceptors licensed their own students to practice. The licensing function then passed to the medical societies and then to the medical schools. But due to abuses and the sorry state of the schools, the state governments finally assumed the licensing function and it continues to be administered by individual state boards of medical examiners today. But this has been less than ideal and many medical educators believe that because of the present supposed uniform quality of medical education today the licensing function should be returned to the schools and the awarding of an M.D. degree should automatically entitle the holder to practice. Such a system would not necessarily do away with the boards of medical examiners as they would presumably investigate the moral qualifications of candidates for licensure. They would also continue to carry out their disciplinary duties.

But, strong as the arguments of the educators appear on the surface, would it really be desirable to turn the licensing duties back to the medical schools? With no intention to express distrust in the integrity of approved schools, my answer is no. In the first place it is desirable to have outside agencies which check on the quality of medical education. The faculty members of many medical schools acknowledge this by voluntarily allowing an outside agency in the form of the National Board of Medical Examiners to evaluate their teaching methods.

In the second place, although the days of the old "C" grade schools are past and we now have only approved schools in the United States, the quality of these schools, as judged by the scores of their graduates on National Board examinations, varies widely. This was emphasized by Hubbard in his study of the graduates of 30 different schools.

How can we best evaluate the curricula of the various medical schools? From a study of the great variety of state medical practice laws it is obvious that the licensing authorities are nowhere near agreement on this. Although no one denies that the examinations of the National Board are of the highest quality, some people who are especially concerned with "states' rights" have an abiding distrust of the organization and either refuse outright to recognize its certificate or grudgingly accept it conditionally. In addition we find that the states are unable to agree on the subjects in which a candidate for licensure should be examined and furthermore there is a wide diversity of passing grades. Yet somehow many states manage to accept the certificates of others for licensure by endorsement. Although the Council of State Governments has long tried to promote uniform licensing laws, its efforts have been in vain and the states continue in their individual ways.

Many boards of medical examiners are in ill repute with both the public and legislatures. They are accused, sometimes unjustly, of fostering monopolies and keeping competition out. In at least two states this criticism is more than justified as the board members freely admit that their examinations are designed not so much to test the knowledge of applicants for licensure but to keep the number of physicians at a level optimal to the establishment. Neither of these states grants licenses by endorsement of the certificate of any other state. One state rigs the grades on a curve, admitting candidates by a quota system so that even those who might have passed the examinations may be given failing grades.

At the opposite extreme we find several states which pass all candidates year after year so that their examinations are worthless and are not trusted by other states.

Another problem is the restriction on movement of physicians within the country through artificial barriers created by lack of endorsement and reciprocity. This difficulty is compounded by the basic science laws, repealed by only three states but still in force in 21 in which these laws constitute another useless hurdle to those wishing to be licensed.

How long will the public continue to tolerate the patchwork of medical practice laws and the capricious restrictions placed upon physicians? This is difficult to answer, but, if sufficiently aroused, the citizens will no doubt eventually rise up in protest. How much better it would be if the states could voluntarily agree upon uniform laws and procedures. After all, this has been almost accomplished in Canada despite the strongly individualistic tendencies of its 12 provinces. Eleven of the 12 accept the certificate of the Medical Council of Canada, the one nonconformist being bilingual Quebec. A possible counterpart of the Medical Council of Canada already exists in this country in the form of the National Board of Medical Examiners, which is continually gaining in stature. Why could not all of the state boards accept diplomates of the National Board for licensure if they met the other requirements of the individual states?

Many of the medical practice laws are so restrictive that they hamper legitimate experiments in medical education. The lockstep system of medical education which served its original purpose to help with the reforms suggested by Flexner, is hopelessly out of date today. But many state laws still cling to the old system of spelling out the medical curriculum in such detail that improvements are well nigh impossible. I am certain the boards of medical examiners and the medical societies can trust the educators not to indulge in wild experimentation merely for the sake of change. Are the state boards so distrustful of the educators that they are unwilling to define the requirement for licensure merely as graduation from an approved school? Everyone concerned from the deans of the medical schools to the most obscure country doctor must realize that many improvements in medical education are necessary and the schools should not be hampered by archaic legal requirements.

Another problem, that of the foreign medical graduate, will no doubt be with us for a long time. While I maintain that in many instances he is being treated unfairly by the licensing boards, there are many responsible educators who say that the requirement of five years of additional training in this country is not too severe. The problem has been compounded by the fact that the Council on Medical Education no longer recognizes any foreign medical schools; this is indeed unfortunate. Therefore the physician from Oxford must be classed with the graduate of the poorest Far Eastern or Latin American school. Why can't the American Medical Association, with its vast resources, extend its interests to include international medical education and again classify foreign medical schools so that the boards of examiners might at least have a guide as to their quality?

The medical examining boards are performing much better in the field of discipline than in education and examination. However, their best efforts are often hampered by the capriciousness of the courts which do not hesitate to substitute their judgement for that of the boards. They often issue stay orders in cases in which the boards have revoked the licenses of physicians. Furthermore, these stay orders permit the defendant to continue his depredations during the long delays before his appeal is finally heard. I suggest that many courts are granting stay orders against the boards entirely too freely and that the situation might be improved if such orders were issued only after a formal preliminary hearing.

The disciplinary functions of the boards are hampered by the fact that they can only act if there has been a violation of the law and this is often difficult to prove because of the reluctance of witnesses to testify and in some instances due to defects in the laws themselves. Therefore the medical profession must often turn to other agencies to protect the public against incompetent, poorly trained physicians. The logical ones are the local medical societies and the hospitals. From the reports of the Department of Medical Ethics of the American Medical Association I judge that the societies are not very active in the field of discipline. The accredited hospitals, with their system of continuous evaluation of patient care by committees, are in a much better position to prevent physicians from carrying out procedures for which they are unqualified. Although no statistical reports on the number and kinds of disciplinary actions taken by hospital staffs are available, their role in this field is assuming ever increasing importance. The boards of medical examiners would do well to work more closely with both the medical societies and the hospital associations.

There is still the problem of the "fringe" hospital which is often the refuge of the unethical and incompetent physicians. California has attempted to solve this problem by placing a passage in its new medical practice law declaring it unethical conduct for a physician to make a habit of practicing in such institutions.

In the field of examining one bright spot has recently appeared with the establishment of the Federation Licensing Examination. This indeed has the potential for the establishment of uniformly high standards throughout the country. It now appears that more boards will adopt it, which is encouraging. A discouraging factor is that already two states, because of the high failure rate of their candidates, have scaled the grades upwards. Let us hope that no more states follow their lead lest this important development come to nought.

To this long-time observer of the medical licensing scene one fault among many stands out. That is the provincialism of the whole system which, based on states' rights, permits

APPENDIX

A Guide to the Essentials of a Modern Medical Practice Act*

INTRODUCTION

The Federation of State Medical Boards of the United States and its members, the individual state and territorial licensing agencies, have recognized the need for a brochure on A Guide to the Essentials of a Modern Medical Practice Act.

Several attempts were made by the Federation to formulate such a brochure until finally at the 1952 Federation meeting, a motion was passed authorizing the appointment of a committee to study The Essentials of a Modern Medical Practice Act. The original committee appointed in 1953 was under the chairmanship of Dr. Bruce Underwood of the Kentucky Board with Dr. Creighton Barker, Connecticut Board; Dr. J. Earl McIntyre, Michigan Board; Dr. Homer Pearson, Florida Board; Dr. S. M. Poindexter, Idaho Board; and Dr. Walter E. Vest, West Virginia Board. In 1954 the same committee was continued, and Dr. George Buck, Colorado Board, was added to the committee. The committee was re-appointed in 1955, but on the resignation of Dr. Bruce Underwood as chairman and as a member, Dr. Buck was appointed chairman.

For the past three years this committee has gathered material. The committee has tried to avoid controversial issues and recommends that individual licensing agencies make additional provisions based on their local circumstances. Brevity has been a foremost consideration.

The recognition of the need for A Guide to the Essentials of a Modern Medical Practice Act by the Federation is confirmed by the work of the committee. This need stems from the study of many medical practice acts which show wide variation in their requirements

* Copyright, 1956, by The Federation of State Medical Boards of the United States. Reprinted by permission. A revision of this document is currently being undertaken, and will probably be completed by the time this book appears. Copies of the revision will be available from Dr. M. H. Crabb, Secretary of the Federation of State Medical Boards of the United States, Suite 304, 1612 Summit Avenue, Ft. Worth, Texas 76102.

and regulations. It is hoped this compendium may serve at least two purposes:

1. To serve as a guide to those states and territories which may adopt a new medical practice act or may be amending existing laws.

2. To encourage standardization of requirements and of regulations to better facilitate reciprocity and endorsement.

A Guide to the Essentials of a Modern Medical Practice Act is intended to serve only as advisory to licensing agencies.

I. Purpose of a Medical Practice Act

A general statement of policy should introduce an act and should emphasize the following facts:

Recognizing that the practice of medicine is a PRIVILEGE granted by legislative authority and is not a NATURAL RIGHT of individuals, it is deemed necessary as a matter of policy in the interests of public health, safety and welfare to provide laws and provisions covering the granting of that privilege and its subsequent use, control and regulation to the end that the public shall be properly protected against unprofessional, improper, unauthorized and unqualified practice of medicine and from unprofessional conduct by persons licensed to practice medicine.

II. Definition

The definition of the practice of medicine may be concisely stated as follows: The practice of medicine by any person shall mean the diagnosis, treatment or correction of, or the attempt to, or the holding of oneself out as being able to diagnose, treat, or correct any and all human conditions, ailments, diseases, injuries or infirmities, whether physical or mental, by any means, method, devices or instrumentalities.

(a) Exceptions to an act:

1. An act should not have application to students who have had training in approved schools of medicine and who are continuing their training and performing the duties of an interne in any hospital or institution maintained and operated by a state or territory or the United States, or in any hospital within a state or territory operating under the supervision of a medical staff, the members of which are licensed to practice medicine and which hospital is approved for internships by a state or territorial licensing agency.

2. An act should not apply to the rendition of service in cases of emergency where no fee or other consideration is charged or received.

3. An act should not be construed to apply to commissioned medical officers of the Armed Forces of the United States, The United States Public Health Service, and medical officers of the Veterans Administration of the United States, in the discharge of their official

duties, nor to licensed physicians from other states or territories if called in consultation with a person licensed to practice medicine.

(b) Exclusions to an act:

The definition of the practice of medicine should not apply to a person licensed to practice a limited field of the healing arts which constitutes a part of the practice of medicine; and the provisions of an act should never be construed to affect in any manner the practice of the religious tenets of any church or religious belief.

III. *Recommendations on Establishment of Licensing Agency or Board and Its Composition*

From ancient times heads of governments and legislative authorities granted to the professions and trades the right to license and regulate their own members. In more modern time, partly due to abuse and partly due to inaction on the part of professions and trades, this privilege has frequently been removed by legislative authority. In many states and territories the authority is vested in non-professional political appointees with professional persons serving without authority and only as advisory. There is a trend to streamline government with the result that licensing boards and agencies are abolished with responsibilities placed in large, multipurpose political departments of government with all authority vested from without the profession. *The medical profession* should insist on the privilege of licensing and regulating its profession with safeguards to protect the public and the individual physician from abuses of privilege.

There should be established in jurisdictional governments an independent board or agency or within an established branch of government, an independent division or board, delegating to it full authority to regulate itself and to carry into effect the provisions of an act. This licensing agency should be allowed full use of funds obtained from licensure fees but under the same regulations applying to other branches of government. The tenure of appointment to the agency should be fixed staggering terms, subject to reappointment and subject to removal *only* when guilty of mal-feasance, mis-feasance or non-feasance.

IV. *Recommendations on Licensure Requirements*

A board should have authority to prescribe and establish rules and regulations to carry into effect provisions of an act including, but without limitation, regulations prescribing all requisite qualifications of education, residence, citizenship, training and character for admission to an examination for licensure.

(a) Minimum requirements should be:

1. That an applicant be at least 21 years of age.
2. That an applicant be of good character.

3. That an applicant be a citizen of the United States.

4. That an applicant graduated from a four-year course of instruction in a medical school or college approved by the licensing agency.

5. That an applicant satisfactorily completed a one-year internship approved by the licensing agency.

6. That an applicant satisfactorily passed the examination required by the licensing agency, unless endorsement or reciprocity procedures are used.

7. That an applicant make a personal appearance before the licensing agency.

(b) Fees should be determined by each licensing agency.

(c) Annual renewals should be required with discretionary authority granted to an agency when the question of competence exists.

V. Examinations

It is recommended that licensing agencies have authority to adopt rules and regulations to:

(a) Prescribe the subjects to be covered in the examination, the number of questions to be asked, the time allowed for answering them, the type of examination (oral or written or both), the method to be used in grading questions, and such other details as may be necessary.

(b) The examination should include questions in the following subjects: Anatomy and its subdivisions; physiology; biochemistry; pathology; bacteriology; pharmacology; medicine; surgery; obstetrics and gynecology; and pediatrics.

(c) Examinations should be given in such a way that persons grading the papers shall have no knowledge of the identity of an individual being examined.

(d) Examinations should be conducted at least semi-annually, provided there are applicants.

(e) A minimum grade in each subject should be 70%; and the minimum general average should be 75%.

VI. Licenses Without Examination

(a) Endorsement: It is recommended that a licensing agency may issue a license by endorsement to an applicant who has complied with licensure requirements and who has passed an examination for a license to practice medicine in all its branches in any other state or territory of the United States, provided that the examination endorsed was, in the opinion of that agency, equivalent in every respect to its examination.

(b) Certifying Agency Examinations: A licensing agency may in its discretion endorse an applicant who has complied with licensure requirements and who has passed an examination given by a recognized certifying agency approved by the licensing agency, provided such examination was, in the opinion of the agency, equivalent in every respect to its examination.

(c) Reciprocity: The licensing agency might in its discretion enter into reciprocal agreements with the licensing agencies of other states or territories providing for the mutual recognition of licenses issued by each state or territory without requiring licentiates to submit to further examination.

(d) Temporary and Special Licenses: It may be desirable to make provision for temporary and special licenses to be in effect in the interval between licensing agency meetings and in order to meet specific needs.

VII. Grounds for Suspension and Revocation of Licenses

To promote more satisfactory endorsement and reciprocity between the several states and territories, mutual understanding on the grounds for suspension and revocation of licenses is necessary.
The Following Charges are Recommended:

1. The use of any false, fraudulent or forged statement or document, or the use of any fraudulent, deceitful, dishonest or immoral practice, in connection with any of the licensing requirements.

2. The performance of an unlawful abortion or assisting or advising the performance of any unlawful abortion.

3. The commission or conviction of a felony.

4. Becoming addicted to a drug or intoxicant to such a degree as to render the licensee unsafe or unfit to practice medicine and surgery.

5. Sustaining any physical or mental disability which renders the further practice of medicine dangerous.

6. The performance of any dishonorable, unethical or unprofessional conduct likely to deceive, defraud or harm the public.

7. The use of any false or fraudulent statement in any document connected with the practice of medicine.

8. Knowingly performing any act which in any way assists an unlicensed person to practice medicine.

9. Violating or attempting to violate, directly or indirectly, or assisting in or abetting the violation of or conspiring to violate any provision or terms of a medical practice act.

10. In case any person holding a license to practice medicine shall by any final order or adjudication of any court of competent jurisdiction be adjudged to be mentally incompetent or insane, the license should automatically be suspended by the licensing agency, and anything in the act to the contrary notwithstanding, such suspension

should continue until the licentiate is found or adjudged by such court to be restored to reason or until he is duly discharged as restored to reason in any other manner provided by law.

11. The practice of medicine under a false or assumed name.

12. The advertising for the practice of medicine in any unethical or unprofessional manner.

13. Obtaining a fee as personal compensation or gain for an employer or for a person on fraudulent representation that a manifestly incurable condition can be permanently cured.

14. The willful violation of privileged communication.

VIII. Definition of Unlawful Practice of Medicine and Violations and Penalties

It should be unlawful for any person to do or perform any act which constitutes the practice of medicine as defined without first having obtained a license to practice medicine.

It is recommended that a person, corporation or association which violates the provisions of a medical practice act or an officer or director of a corporation or association causing or aiding and abetting such violation, shall be deemed guilty of a felony, and upon conviction thereof shall be punished by imprisonment for a term not exceeding two years or by a fine not exceeding $1000.00 or by both such fine and imprisonment.

IX. Proceedings for Revocation and Suspension

It is recommended that a procedure be enacted placing full authority in a licensing agency. An agency should have discretion concerning probation, suspension and revocation. The findings of an agency should be subject to review by courts, but the courts' authority should be limited to sustain or reverse a decision, not to modify.

X. Injunction Clause

Such a clause is recommended to institute proceedings against unlawful practice. An agency should maintain a suit for injunction against any person, corporation or association and the officers and directors of any such corporation or association, violating the provisions of a medical practice act. Any such person, corporation or association and the officers and directors thereof so enjoined should be punished for contempt for violation of such injunction by the court issuing the same. An injunction should be issued without proof of actual damage sustained by any person. An injunction should not relieve a person, corporation or association, nor the officers or directors thereof from criminal prosecution for violation of the Medical Practice Act.

XI. *Rules and Regulations to be Adopted by Licensing Agency*

A Medical Practice Act should authorize each licensing agency to adopt rules and regulations to carry into effect the provisions of its medical practice act.

INDEX

Abortion, criminal, 78
Addiction:
  as manifestation of mental illness, 82
  as occupational disease, 81
  depression as cause of, 82
  of physicians to narcotics, 78
Addicts
  personality type of, 82
  rehabilitation of, 83
  varying rates of relapse in, 81
Alcoholism, 78
American Academy of General Practice, 16
American Board of Neurological Surgery. *See* National Board of Medical Examiners
American College of Physicians: self-evaluation program of, 16
American Confederation of Reciprocating Examining and Licensing Medical Boards, 49
American Hospital Association: and cooperation with Department of Investigation, 116
American Medical Association
and licensing function of schools, 11
approval of National Board, 63
disciplinary committee of, 89
Disciplinary Digest of, 93
efforts at improvement of medical education, 49
financial support of Federation by, 58
influence on educational standards, 6
influence on medical licensure, 28
interest in incompetence, 87

support of a national board of medical examiners, 62
support of national examining board, 50
American Medical Association, Congress on Medical Education integration with programs of Federation, 54
American Medical Association, Council on Medical Education accredited foreign medical schools, 139
endorsement of national board, 63
interest in Federation, 50
American Medical Association, Department of Investigation, 106, 115, 116
American Medical Association, Judicial Council of: jurisdiction of, 89
American Medical Eclectic College of Cincinnati, 15
Amphetamines, illegal sale of, 78
Appel, James Z., 87
Apprentice system, 3
Arizona, revised medical practice laws of, 25
Arkansas State Eclectic Medical Board of Examiners, 51
Arkansas, State Medical Board of the Arkansas Medical Society, 52
Association of American Medical Colleges
influence on medical licensure, 28
interest in National Confederation, 50
jointly sponsored meetings with Federation, 54

177

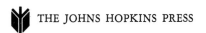 THE JOHNS HOPKINS PRESS

Designed by Edward D. King

*Composed in American Garamond text
by Baltimore Type and Composition Corporation*

*Printed on 60-lb. Perkins and Squier R
by Universal Lithographers, Inc.*

*Bound in Interlaken Vellum, AV 3-975
by The Maple Press Company*